HELP YOURSELF TO MENTAL HEALTH

Also by Mary Manning

The Drugs Menace

HELP YOURSELF TO MENTAL HEALTH

Mary Manning

COLUMBUS BOOKS
LONDON

First published in Great Britain in 1988 by
Columbus Books Limited
19-23 Ludgate Hill
London EC4M 7PD

For Patricia, Anne and Christine

British Library Cataloguing in Publication Data
Manning, Mary
  Help yourself to mental health
    1. Women – Mental health
    I. Title
    613'.Q4244   RC451.4.W6
    ISBN 0-86287-341-X

Typeset in Palatino by Facet Film Composing Limited,
Leigh-on-Sea, Essex.

Printed and bound by The Guernsey Press, Guernsey, CI.

Contents

Introduction

What do we mean by mental health? Do we see it as a state of mental well-being which we take for granted when we are feeling happy and 'in control'? Or do we see it as implying freedom from psychiatric disorder? Do we shy away from the very thought of mental health because we perceive in the term some vaguely disquieting threat of breakdown or madness? It is a fact that we seldom see the term 'mental health' used other than in the context of breakdown and, more specifically, of psychotic illness, in which the sufferer becomes mentally confused and temporarily loses touch with reality.

Yet the fact is that severe disorders of this kind are relatively rare compared with the much more common complaints that come under the general heading of neurotic illness: anxiety, depression, eating and drinking disorders and phobias. Because these problems spring largely from attitudes and thought patterns which are more open to self-assessment and more amenable to change through the medium of self-help, these are the areas on which this book focuses most of its attention.

It is estimated that in Britain about one woman in every six or seven, and one man in every nine or ten, will need to seek medical help for some psychological complaint at some time. One-third of all family doctor consultations now involve some element of psychological problem although, more often than not, the declared purpose of the patient's visit may be to discuss a physical problem: most of us still find it easier to talk about physical pain than to say we are feeling depressed. But while most emotionally ill patients seen by GPs are successfully treated without having to be referred to a psychiatrist, there are likely to be many more sufferers who never see a doctor or therapist;

they are the ones who recover spontaneously – or reach the point of total breakdown.

Differences between the sexes in terms of vulnerability to psychological problems are of special interest to researchers. Although women tend to live longer than men, they seem much more susceptible to neurotic illness. On the other hand, men are just as likely to be affected by a condition such as schizophrenia, which is believed to be rooted in some disturbance of brain chemistry. One explanation for gender differences in reported cases of emotional distress may be that where it is possible to conceal this, men usually manage to do so, since in most societies it is seen as weak and unmanly to admit to such a feeling. Because of conditioning in our society, men are much readier to use alcohol as a tranquillizer than to ask the doctor for help. And when their problems become too much for them to bear, they are more likely to take their own lives. Women are generally more ready to seek help and accept treatment, and to try to understand the causes of their problems. A woman is more likely to make an unsuccessful suicide attempt which might be interpreted as a cry for help. The clarification of factors leading to apparently greater mental ill-health in women has been one of the major contributions of the women's movement: social and environmental pressures particularly predispose women to severe depression.

Despite the advances made in understanding psychological disorders in recent times, the stigma of mental illness still persists to some extent. As a result, we may deny ourselves helpful treatment rather than risk being labelled as disturbed or neurotic or as someone who is 'seeing a psychiatrist' and is therefore having 'serious problems'. So concerned was the American Psychiatric Association about the ill-effects of such labelling that in 1980 it decided to abolish the term 'neurosis' when compiling a revised classification of mental disorders. In Britain, the term has been retained on the grounds that it provides a more convenient method of classifying a particular range of problems than the various alternatives suggested.

In everyday language, however, we tend to use the

familiar term 'emotional problems' to distinguish neurotic disorders, which are mainly concerned with feelings, from more severe mental illnesses involving disturbances of thought.

It is rare for people suffering from neurotic illnesses to need in-patient hospital care: only a tiny proportion of psychiatric hospital beds are occupied by patients who have these problems, whereas admission to hospital is common for patients suffering from psychotic illnesses.

The main differences between neurotic and psychotic illnesses are that in neurosis contact with reality is retained, whereas in psychosis it is lost for the time being; in neurosis only part of the personality is affected, while psychosis involves the whole personality; in neurosis behaviour is related to the sufferer's usual personality, whereas psychosis involves a change of personality; neurosis often results from stress, but psychosis may have no apparent 'triggering' cause.

Almost half of all psychiatric hospital beds are occupied by schizophrenia patients. About one-eighth are occupied by sufferers from manic-depressive psychosis, and a further one-eighth by sufferers from dementia, a condition due to a form of brain damage which affects some older people. However, largely because of the effectiveness of modern drugs in altering and shortening the course of many of these more severe disorders, the time which most patients now spend in hospital has been reduced dramatically – usually to months rather than years, as was once the case.

While recent times have seen many improvements in the treatment of more serious mental disorders, a great deal remains to be done in terms of providing desperately needed accommodation and support in the community for chronically ill patients and their families. A great deal also needs to be done for the many other mentally ill people permanently resident in our prisons because suitable alternative care cannot be found for them. We can all help by supporting campaigns designed to influence social policy at a national level, and by taking an interest in the efforts being made by our own local authorities to honour their statutory obligations for the welfare of mentally ill people. By helping others we can also help ourselves to overcome those feelings of helplessness, isolation and personal frustration which contribute to lesser degrees of mental ill-health.

We are much more fortunate than our forebears in that today it is acceptable to admit to feelings of misery, anxiety and depression, and that there is so much help available if we know where to look for it. We are lucky also to live at a time when professionals are much more interested in learning about these problems and in finding effective ways of treating them rather than adopting dismissive attitudes towards complaints that are very real to us.

Because women are still the majority of sufferers from these complaints and because they are still the people likely to take most interest in the well-being of their families and their menfolk, this book is primarily addressed to them. In it I have set out to explain the background to the common ailments to which any one of us may be prone at some time, and to show what we can do to help ourselves in terms of clearer understanding, prevention and self-help. At the same time I wish to interpret 'self-help' in its broadest sense by emphasizing the importance of seeking medical help when needed, and the benefit to be gained from the sensible use of prescribed therapeutic drugs in helping to relieve distress and restore equilibrium. Equally, I want to stress the value of mutual help groups and professional counselling and psychotherapy, especially as alternatives to repeat prescriptions for anti-depressants and tranquillizers.

Although I write partly from experience gained as a nurse working with people suffering from emotional problems and more serious forms of mental illness, and partly from experience gained as a medical journalist and counsellor with a special interest in mental health, I feel that by far my most important qualification for venturing on this task is the understanding gained through having been a fellow-sufferer. One lesson I have learned personally is that there is a close relationship between anxiety, depression, panic and phobic attacks – that for most of us they are all part of the same pattern of neurotic response to social pressures. Another is that a sympathetic doctor, appropriate medication and a supportive family can go a long way towards reassuring the sufferer that there is light at the end of the tunnel.

CHAPTER 1

Women and depression

We all tend to feel depressed from time to time, and often for no particular reason. This is something we learn to live with, knowing that the bleak mood will soon pass and the sun will shine again. Most of us are familiar with early morning 'blues' which evaporate quite magically once we are up and about. Mood changes throughout the day are quite common, probably depending to a large extent on the workings of the internal 'biological clocks' which regulate our chemical functions. Variations in the weather, too, can have a marked effect on mood, of course, and – as if we didn't know it already – studies have revealed that people living in cooler climates feel happier and more purposeful on sunny days.

Depression is not the same thing as unhappiness. The latter is something we have learnt to live with as we grew up, unless we were exceptionally fortunate indeed. Being unhappy or 'feeling depressed' temporarily are common experiences which we don't normally allow to interfere with our responsibilities and general routine. An obvious sign that we may be about to cross the dividing line leading to 'clinical depression' and an urgent need for treatment is that our sadness and self-absorption are interfering with our work and relationships. If this feeling continues day after day, then it is time to seek help.

However, the onset of severe depression often is so insidious that the sufferer is aware only of feeling increasingly miserable and lifeless. Assuming that she must be 'run-down' physically, she may buy vitamin supplements from the chemist. If these don't seem to help, she may pay a visit to the doctor, without ever mentioning that she feels depressed. Young mothers and older married women who are at home all day are particularly prone to depression. Even in the most stable marriages, women confined to the home day after day often tend to find their isolation burdensome, without anyone being aware of their need for adult company. They miss the companionship and interests which they previously found in their employment and, at the same time, they feel guilty about not being able to derive total satisfaction from the roles of wife and mother. If they have no friends or close relatives living near at hand, or if they have a partner who spends many of his evenings away from home too, then their lives can be very lonely indeed. Despite growing concern in sociological circles about the effects of family breakdown, the wisdom of the high-rise residential block phenomenon, and especially the life style of young house-bound mothers, the mental health of working-class women was a subject that attracted little attention even 20 years ago.

But is it really true that women are more prone to depression than men? Is this apparent trend not merely a reflection of women's greater readiness to admit to emotional 'weakness' and to make more use of the health services? This is a proposition which has attracted a considerable amount of medical and sociological research in recent years. And, yes, it does appear to be true that – all things being equal – women are generally more susceptible to severe forms of depression. Where studies show an increasing incidence of depression among men, this tends to be among the long-term unemployed, among those thrust unexpectedly into early retirement, and younger men enduring a long wait before they can even begin earning a living. In other words, men tend to respond in much the same way as women to similar precipitating factors; and their conditioning may make it even less easy for them to tolerate loneliness and disappointment.

While the greater vulnerability of women to depression may be considered an accepted fact, controversy continues to flourish with regard to its cause. What differences of opinion boil down to is a fresh slant on the old argument of nature versus nurture as the main root of the problem.

On the one hand there are those – mainly doctors – who insist that fluctuations in hormone levels throughout the

13

menstrual cycle and at the menopause play a prominent role in the emotional well-being of women. Where this association can be confirmed, it is claimed that the best approach is to correct the imbalance by giving synthetic hormones as treatment.

On the other hand, the sociological explanation is that women are much more likely to become depressed through the crushing influence of environmental factors like loneliness, material deprivation, financial worries, bad housing conditions, lack of personal achievement, and the absence of a close, confiding relationship, ideally with a sexual partner. Even with such a stressful background, a woman will often survive without developing a full-blown clinical depression until she encounters some calamitous 'life event' such as loss of a relationship, loss of hope of rehousing and so on, which tips the balance.

George W. Brown and Tirril Harris, respectively as professor of sociology and research officer at Bedford College, London, studied large numbers of women over a long period in the mid-1970s. As a result, they were able to identify four factors which seemed to enhance the depressive effects of disturbing life events and major difficulties. These were: that the woman had lost her mother through death or long-term separation before she reached the age of eleven; that she had three or more children under the age of fourteen living with her; that she did not have a full-time or part-time job outside the home; and that she did not have someone such as a husband, boyfriend or close relative in whom she could confide.

The researchers found that only further, more serious life events with lasting implications were likely to trigger an attack of depression. These included separation or the threat of it through desertion or death; life-threatening illness in someone close; an unpleasant revelation about someone close, such as a partner's infidelity, which called for a complete reassessment of the relationship; the threat of substantial material loss or disappointment, relating to issues like housing and unemployment; and persistent marital difficulties.

The average age of women with this type of reactive

depression (see page 21) in the study was 29. For the much smaller number of women found with non-reactive depression the average age was 45, which is in accord with medical experience generally. Just over a quarter of severely depressed middle-class women, and nearly half of depressed working-class women, did not have a husband or boyfriend with whom they could share their anxieties. It was observed that poor living conditions and poor relationships predisposed to depression and also inhibited women against seeking medical advice once they reached the point where help was urgently needed.

Because low self-esteem and feelings of inadequacy, unworthiness and guilt are such common features of clinical depression, it has sometimes been suggested that these manifestations add up to evidence of a 'depression-prone personality' rooted either in a biological predisposition, or in some damaging emotional experience in early childhood. No evidence has been found to support this demoralizing argument, which suggests that being a 'depressive' is a more or less inescapable state of mind for some sufferers. Brown and Harris point out that 'There is no justification at all for giving priority to hereditary or constitutional factors.' Vulnerability to life-events can result exclusively from a deleterious social environment.

Just as importantly, it is argued that women with poor self-esteem may find it difficult to establish and maintain good personal relationships of the kind needed for support in times of trouble and doubt. They may even end up choosing partners who themselves find it difficult to enter into a confiding relationship, because they have lost hope of finding a more loving and supportive partner who would accept them. It is said that while men blame others for their depression, women tend to blame themselves. This certainly seems to be true of many women who say they stay in an unhappy relationship for the most negative reasons. 'He accepts me – I don't think anyone else would put up with me,' I was told by one young woman who might otherwise be envied for her good looks, intelligence and qualifications.

Being happily married – as far as outward appearances

are concerned – is no guarantee that the couple's relationship really is a supportive and confiding one. On the contrary, many seemingly well-adjusted couples seldom discuss personal or financial problems, which is one good reason for involving marriage guidance counsellors in more GPs' surgeries on an 'attachment' basis.

'We are all conditioned to taking a very lop-sided view of marriage,' says Joan, a social worker. 'There is a general impression that all you need for a good relationship is sexual compatibility – that the so-called sexual chemistry is some sort of a magical ingredient which can put everything else right. In fact, it is the other way round – when the sexual relationship starts going wrong it is more likely to be because other pressures of everyday life are getting in the way. For instance, it is very difficult for a woman to switch over to being cosy and romantic at a given time, when she is really feeling quite resentful about many of the practical problems for which she feels she has to take an unequal share of responsibility.

'Women hate being dependent on men for money, for example. This dependence has always been the case in households where income is limited, and wives have had to be accountable for stretching their share of a man's wages as far as possible. I grew up in a working-class home with really good, hard-working parents, and I know my own mother was always worrying about shortage of money and wishing she could get 'a wee part-time job', as she described it . . . The fact is that there are no-go areas in far too many partnerships, and discussion about cash problems and work-sharing in housework and child care are among the most important of these. How can you have a confiding relationship if you're with someone who just doesn't want to know anything about the practicalities of managing a home on a very low cash allowance?'

However, another perhaps even more important cause of disappointment and depression among married women is lack of affection in the relationship, according to Penny, a marriage guidance counsellor.

'Not nearly enough attention is paid to what women

themselves say they want from a relationship, and they have been saying quite a lot over the past ten years or so. In marriage counselling, we see one side of the lives of women whose marriages run into problems, and a great deal of what we see is remarkably consistent with what women say in their writings, and in the information which comes out of the sort of attitude surveys conducted by women's magazines and the like.

'It's a pity that such surveys tend to be dismissed by the orthodox research establishment, on the grounds that participants are self-selected, or that the study's methodology doesn't measure up to the demands of sociological criteria, and so forth. So you will seldom see them quoted anywhere. Yet they often reflect women's true feelings very clearly. And what so many of them seem to be saying is that they can tolerate all sorts of hardship in a relationship, provided it is one in which there is affection and trust and fair play.

'They see a loving relationship as being one in which there is warmth and closeness, and displays of affection occur spontaneously without necessarily having sexual overtones. In fact, women become very disenchanted with men who never show affection except as a prelude to intercourse.

'Men can be very uptight about demonstrations of affection. They are conditioned from an early age to regard such displays as weakness – something they could never admit to needing themselves. In a world obsessed with sexual prowess and being "good in bed" – however this is to be interpreted – there is no-one to tell them that the real key to a loving relationship is tenderness and the spontaneous little gestures which say so much more than words.

'If we are able to talk to both partners, we often can do a lot to bridge the gap, but women themselves find it difficult to break down this sort of reserve. Besides, they feel that any show of affection which has to be asked for isn't worth having and may not be genuine. And, during courtship the relationship may have been very different. My feeling about many so-called promiscuous women is that they are

17

constantly searching for something which they have found unattainable in a stable relationship – and it's rarely sexual satisfaction. As a result, they feel they are selling themselves short and get depressed.'

Research has shown that married women, especially those who don't go out to work, are more prone to depression than people in all other groups. On the other hand, married men are much less susceptible than single, divorced and widowed men and women. This finding suggests that the average man finds in marriage something which is not available to women – a support structure which buffers him against the stresses of everyday life while allowing him to enjoy job-satisfaction and many of the interests of his bachelor days. The increased vulnerability of married women is attributed to lack of social contacts and economic independence, and the poor self-esteem associated with the low status of child care and housework. It was interesting to hear Professor Anthony Clare's summing-up of the consistent global view of marriage gained through a world-wide investigation for the BBC2 television series *Lovelaw*: in every society explored it was found that men, having originally established the ground-rules for marriage as a power-base, invariably got the best deal from marriage and women came out a poor second.

Going out to work seldom offers women a complete solution, however. On the contrary, that too can often be a demoralizing experience. It usually involves the dual responsibility of combining a job with running a home. Many women can find work only in underpaid jobs with no prospect of advancement. Even in jobs where promotion is on the cards, competent women may find themselves repeatedly passed over in favour of men with fewer qualifications.

Sexual harassment can take many forms, and the most crudely distasteful forms are not always the ones which hurt most, says Sue, an experienced medical secretary aged 35. Her worst moment came after she had applied for a senior job in a major teaching hospital.

'The vacancy was in a specialty in which I had a particular

interest and I would have been working for a top consultant. So I was very keen to get the post and felt confident about applying for it. Then came the day of the interview, and I'm sitting waiting in the reception area of the hospital when the great man dashes in from somewhere and calls out to the clerk at the inquiries desk: "I'm expecting a little girl for interview. Give me a call when she arrives." And he looked right through me as if I couldn't possibly be the applicant.' We live in a society where women are constantly being assessed by men in terms of age and appearance; consequently, this is an extremely sensitive emotional minefield for many women.

While there is no doubt that men who suffer from depression also experience feelings of failure and worthlessness and guilt, it seems particularly significant that these emotions tend to be such a prominent feature of depression among women. The traditional romantic view of feminine happiness and well-being is that of an eminently fair and dutiful young lady, basking contentedly in the sunshine of her lord's esteem. In a radically altered world where almost everything else has changed, many women still see their worth as being defined very largely in terms of masculine appreciation and of those early values.

There can be no doubt that much of the guilt and self-doubt which most women experience at some time is rooted in early educational conditioning, especially with regard to sexual morality, and in what has amounted to an inherent sense of inferiority fostered by leaders of men throughout the ages from St Augustine to Martin Luther down to our own age.

SYMPTOMS OF DEPRESSION

The symptoms of depression can vary considerably, according to the severity of the illness and the type of depression involved. Needless to say, not everyone who is depressed is likely to experience all of the symptoms listed here. Some people will have suffered from a number simultaneously or at different times. Very often, a depressed person finds it difficult to describe 'negative' attitudes until prompted by a checklist of this kind.

- Tiredness, listlessness, lacking energy
- Anxiety, irritability, easily agitated
- Not interested in usual activities
- Increasing worry about physical health
- Frequent weeping and feelings of sadness
- Relationships with others deteriorating
- Loss of appetite or overeating
- Marked weight loss or rapid weight-gain
- Loss of self-confidence
- Deteriorating self-image
- Loss of interest in home and appearance
- Insomnia, especially in early morning
- Loss of interest, or increased interest, in sex
- Dependence on alcohol, drugs, gambling, etc.
- Anti-social behaviour, such as shoplifting
- Inability to concentrate or make decisions
- Feelings of guilt and unworthiness
- Feeling that memory is impaired
- Slowness in thought and movement
- Fear of being left alone or dying
- Frequent suicidal thoughts

CHAPTER 2

Types of depression

When someone is suffering from severe or long-standing depression, discovering the nature of the illness can be very important, because on that depend treatment and prevention of further episodes. Because so many symptoms are common to most types, establishing the true diagnosis is often a gradual process occurring over several months. So it helps if the sufferer can give as much information as possible about the illness. For diagnostic purposes, doctors use certain broad classifications to distinguish between the different types of depression. These include:

reactive
endogenous
manic-depression
masked depression
depression due to or associated with physical illness
depression due to drugs
depression in old age
seasonal affective disorder
post-natal depression (see pages 54-55).

The following descriptions include some examples of the different types.

REACTIVE DEPRESSION
Often called the 'common cold of psychiatry', this type is by far the most prevalent and easiest to diagnose. It is regarded as essentially self-limiting, and many patients recover in time without treatment. Studies have shown that the illness is a reaction to social pressures like loneliness, isolation, poverty, lack of achievement and dissatisfaction with life in general; and that it can develop as a gradual downhill process unnoticed by relatives and friends.

Usually it tends to come to a head when triggered by some traumatic 'life event'. This may be something as shattering as a sudden bereavement, the break-up of a relationship, or the blighting of hopes for a career; but sometimes the 'last straw' for someone already vulnerable may seem relatively trivial to observers.

Like many young mothers in a stressful situation, Frances concealed her own feelings as best she could. As a divorced mother with two children under school age, her opportunities for making friends were limited. Still shocked and bewildered over the break-up of her marriage and the loss of her home, she kept asking herself where had she gone wrong. Because she could not come to terms with her plight as an unsupported single parent, and was new to her present neighbourhood, she had not contacted any of the local self-help groups which might have provided moral and material support. Besides, she found her situation so painful and humiliating that she could not bear to discuss it with anyone except her sister, who lived abroad.

Living on the third floor of a decaying tenement which was due for demolition, and with only social security payments on which to keep herself and the children, Frances' living environment and daily routine certainly had all the ingredients conducive to depressive breakdown. Yet she managed to keep afloat, as so many others do in similar circumstances, until one further shattering 'life event' occurred – she heard that her sister had been seriously injured in a road accident. Even then it was several months later before she finally felt desperately in need of help, and decided to consult her GP.

'I didn't know where to turn. Then I thought that at least I was entitled to go to the doctor and ask for something to calm my nerves. By this time I couldn't eat or sleep or stop thinking about how hopeless everything was and that I might never see my sister again. It troubled me a lot that I couldn't even visit her in hospital, and that if she survived she was likely to end up paralysed. Fortunately, this turned out not to be the case, but I had no way of knowing this at the time.

'At that time I was also afraid that my social security would be stopped because an official had called not long before this, asking a lot of questions and looking around the place very pointedly. Maybe it was just a routine visit, but you get a bit paranoid when you're living on social security. I thought, "They think I'm cohabiting with some man and that he should be supporting us." I'd never even had a boyfriend at this stage, but it suddenly seemed grossly unfair that I couldn't have a relationship without risking our only income. As it happened, I needn't have worried, but that visit made me feel more boxed in than ever with no prospect of a life of my own. By the way, I still think it's a monstrous idea that if a single mother has a boyfriend who occasionally stays overnight, he is assumed to be supporting her and her children!'

Frances found that her visit to the doctor was a more positive step than she could have anticipated.

'I'm afraid I didn't expect much help as I'd heard so much about doctors being unsympathetic. So I just said my piece about having no appetite and not sleeping and feeling depressed, thinking that she would just write a prescription for anti-depressants and I would go away. But before giving me a prescription she asked a lot of questions about my health and my personal circumstances, and the result was that I lost control and burst into tears and found myself blurting out the whole story. I think it was her kindness that got to me, because I couldn't stop crying. She said not to worry when I apologized for taking up so much time. I still cry when I remember it.

'Anyway, I did get a lot of help afterwards. The doctor arranged for a health visitor and social worker to visit me, and they were able to introduce me to a self-help group and a playgroup for the children, which I took my turn in helping to run, along with other parents. The social worker was very helpful with practical problems, and in talking about the various aspects of my situation, so that in time I could stop blaming myself for our troubles. She explained that every deserted wife feels rejected, and that when people feel rejected it is not unusual for them to think it's because they don't deserve better treatment, and that there is something lacking in themselves. I know that being able to talk to other single mothers – most of them divorced or separated – helped a lot to put my own experience into perspective. In fact, I was surprised to find so many women who had been through the same sort of experience. It was also a revelation to discover how much women can do to help each other when they combine forces. For instance, one group had organized a baby-sitting circle so that we could take it in turns to have an evening out. It certainly has meant a lot to me.

'So if I were asked to advise someone who is at the stage which I had reached a few years ago, the first thing I would say is: Don't bottle it up as I did. Don't lock yourself away so that nobody knows you're even there. Don't blame yourself for whatever has happened in the past – it's a waste of time and emotion anyway. Above all, don't wait until you're really falling apart before seeking help. There probably is a lot going on in your neighbourhood to help people with all sorts of problems, if you would only look. If you don't you'll never know how much friendship there is out there for the asking. The tragedy is that so many people, like myself, have to be at the end of their tether to find out about it.'

It certainly is arguable that the so-called permissive revolution which did so much to liberate women from the burden of unwanted childbearing also went much further in liberating men from their share of responsibility in sexual relationships. This is the view expressed by Angela, who grew up in a very religious family, and attributes her recent breakdown and hospitalization to an abortion which she had nearly thirteen years earlier when she was eighteen.

'There really wasn't anything else I could have done at the time. I do see that but being rational about it doesn't seem to make much difference to the way I feel. Richard and I were both at university, and my pregnancy resulted from carelessness on my part, because it was taken for granted that contraception was my responsibility. I didn't mind that at all at the time. It's only lately that I have become resentful about my being the one to be responsible and having to suffer all the agonising involved in a termination, and the guilt and sense of loss which followed much later. In an odd sort of way I think the memory would have been less painful if I had eventually married someone else who wasn't involved. I've been married to Richard for over ten years now and we have a wonderful daughter, but I'm convinced that he has never given a moment's thought to that other child which he encouraged me to destroy, who would have been about twelve now, had he been allowed to live. I always think of that baby as having been a boy, although I have no knowledge to base this assumption on, of course.

'What Richard said after the operation at a Birmingham nursing home was, "Great! Now the thing to do is to forget you ever were here, so let's not talk about it any more." I was vastly relieved that I had finally agreed to go through with the abortion after a lot of heart-searching and deception, to prevent my parents from finding out about it, because the alternatives were too devastating. But I had been through a major emotional and physical experience, and I did want to talk about it. In fact, we never did discuss it. Perhaps the main reason for this was that Richard felt badly about it too, as my psychiatrist suggested years later. I only know that he got terribly angry when, one day in the depths of depression, I reminded him that our "son" would now have been ten years old. "You're sick – really sick!" he yelled at me. And that was the only time we ever spoke about it.

'I didn't deliberately set out to think about the abortion. It just kept sneaking back into my mind at odd moments at first, some time after we had discussed having another baby and Richard was so much against it that I finally accepted his arguments. I would suddenly see a boy of the same age as our child, had he lived. Or I might be looking at our daughter, and completely out of the "blue" a shadowy figure would appear behind her like a ghost. Then this sort of thing was happening more and more often, and I was getting more depressed and guilt-ridden, and there was nobody I could confide in. At the same time, I realised that I was being very unfair to my husband and daughter, which only made me feel even more guilty and grief-stricken.

'The awful thing was that nothing could be done to change matters. There was no way that I could undo the decision I had taken ten years before. In my calmer moments I realised that I was becoming quite paranoid, to say the least, but I couldn't get the past out of my mind. When I finally agreed to see a psychiatrist I still couldn't talk about the loss which was uppermost in my mind. After a while I found I could talk to a psychotherapist who spent quite a lot of time with me when I was admitted to a private hospital. She went into my background quite a lot, and one day when I thought she seemed to be floundering about looking for a cause of my illness in my relationship with my parents, I got exasperated and I said I knew precisely why I was ill and I explained what had been happening.

'Even then, she seemed to think that my reaction to the abortion had a lot to do with my religious upbringing, and my feelings about what the attitude of my parents would have been, had they known about it. Although I still held to my Catholic beliefs I had not been to church for years, and I had never confessed to a priest since the termination. I often wished that I could, but it's not something you can do easily. I couldn't see myself kneeling in a dark confessional to tell a strange priest that I had been in a state of mortal sin for years, and now could he please give me absolution so that I could feel better about it, knowing that God had forgiven me. It seemed very much like hypocrisy to me.

'As the psychotherapist wasn't a Christian, I was surprised when she advised me to go to confession. She said: "Maybe if you thought that God had forgiven you, you might begin to forgive yourself. And perhaps your religion could help you to accept that what is done cannot be undone, but that learning to live with pain may be a basis for emotional and spiritual growth." When I explained my objection about confessing to a strange priest, she made inquiries and surprised me further by coming up with the name of an understanding priest who was also involved in running a mental health self-help group. For me, this introduction proved to be the turning point, and perhaps there are others who could be helped in the same way.

'Of course, this experience left me wondering whether I had been suffering from an illness of the mind or of the spirit. So I put the question to my therapist when I went for my last appointment. She said it's impossible to distinguish between mind and soul on clinical grounds, and that we all have a spiritual element in our make-up which can be expressed through art and music and great literature as well as through religion. While she was sure that many people found solace in religion and that not enough attention was paid to this aspect of spirituality in modern society, she also felt that religion can in itself sometimes have a damaging effect, especially where its teaching places a lot of emphasis on sin and guilt at an early age, which can amount to a form of "conditioning".

'In modern life it could be difficult for a young person to maintain the sort of standards required of them, she said. And if they took their moral training very seriously, or if they were vulnerable in some way through an inherited weakness, then they could find themselves in trouble when things went wrong. She certainly implied that something like this had happened in my case. So I'm willing to accept that, while for me religion certainly was part of the cure, it may also have contributed to the guilt.'

Reactive depression can have many symptoms in common with other types. Where it tends to differ from its near neighbour – endogenous depression – is that patients are less likely to complain of loss of appetite, physical ailments, or early morning waking. Where there are sleeping problems, these tend to involve difficulty in getting to sleep and disturbed sleep during the night. Sufferers do tend to lose their self-confidence and to blame themselves for their misfortunes. Medical treatment for reactive depression may include drugs such as tricyclic anti-depressants and drugs in the MAOI group: 'monoamine oxidase inhibitors' (see page 142). For someone with a deep-seated or long-standing problem, psychotherapy can be recommended, either on an individual or group basis. However, facilities for psychotherapy under the NHS tend to vary considerably throughout the country; and private psychotherapy can also be scarce in in many areas, as well as being expensive. Cognitive therapy, which aims to change harmful ways of thinking, is being used increasingly where services are available, and it is also being incorporated into the work of self-help groups which have a therapy element in their meetings.

ENDOGENOUS DEPRESSION
Sometimes described as 'true depression', this can also be triggered by some distressing 'life event', but it is regarded essentially as 'coming from within' the sufferer's own mind, due to disturbances in brain chemistry which may have a genetic component. Early morning waking with very severe depression which lessens during the day is one of the main symptoms of this type of depression (see page 147). Physical complaints and loss of appetite are also frequent characteristics.

Treatment can include drugs used for reactive depression. Where these fail to provide help after a reasonable period, the patient may be offered ECT (electro-convulsive therapy) or lithium may be prescribed in some severe cases. A newer approach pioneered in the United States is artificial daylight treatment, which is used mainly for seasonal affective disorder (see page 49). Psychotherapy is found to be less helpful, because obviously it is less easy to influence thinking and behaviour through 'talking treatment' where the problem is believed to have a physical cause.

When someone becomes profoundly depressed for no apparent reason, and especially if another member of the family has had a similar illness, a doctor is likely to consider the possibility of endogenous depression. But before making a firm diagnosis on the assumption that there may be an inherited predisposition to this type of depression, other factors have to be weighed up. There is the probability that everyone in the family shares to some extent social pressures which may equally well predispose to reactive depression. Whatever the type, depression always tends to be associated with some disruption of the sufferer's lifestyle and relationships. In reactive depression, disruption and a sense of losing control usually precede the illness, whereas in endogenous depression the illness is more likely to come first. However, by the time someone decides to seek medical advice, such fine distinctions are unlikely to be remembered. But if some recent research proves as promising as doctors hope, it may be possible soon to have a blood test capable of identifying endogenous depression.

The feasibility of such a blood test was described by Professor Brian Leonard of Galway University at a recent conference. This possibility is an extension of continuing research into the question of a direct relationship between endogenous depression and disturbances in the delicate biochemistry of the brain and central nervous system. Studies have concentrated on the role of neurotransmitters, the chemicals which facilitate the transmission of electrical impulses between the nerve cells which govern all human activity, including our thoughts, moods and movements. Although a great deal has still to be learnt about these recently discovered chemicals, it is believed that they hold the key to treatment and to the manner in which ECT and drugs like anti-depressants achieve beneficial effects.

Of the 40 or more neurotransmitters already known, two have been singled out as being particularly important in the study of depression: noradrenaline and serotonin. Both of these have been found to be functioning well below the normal level in depressed patients. More recent research has shown that certain blood cells (the platelets which are concerned with clotting) have receptors similar to those in the central nervous system, which take up these chemicals. Serotonin uptake by these blood cells is found to be reduced in endogenous depression, but not in reactive depression. Moreover, serotonin uptake has been found to return to the normal level once the depression is relieved. Considerably more research needs to be done, however, before this discovery is likely to lead to a simple blood test capable of identifying endogenous depression in the initial stages.

MANIC DEPRESSION
Called 'hypomania' in mild cases and 'manic-depressive

psychosis' in more severe cases. This is an illness in which, as the name suggests, long periods of depression alternate with 'manic' phases, during which the sufferer feels highly elated, over-optimistic about the future, and engages in frenetic activity of one kind or another. A person in the manic phase may lose contact with reality to an extent where he or she sees the world through the proverbial rose-coloured glasses, for the time being at least. Debts can be accumulated, extravagant purchases made, and chaos can result, if the condition is not recognized and treated.

Because of its alternating swings of mood from elation and super-charged energy to crushing despair, manic depression has tended to be identified with creative genius in the retrospective view of some modern medical observers. It is said that the nineteenth-century composer, Schumann, conceived his greatest work during the 'high' phase; during a 'low' phase of overwhelming depression he threw himself into the Rhine. Other composers, such as Elgar, Handel, Rachmaninov and Wagner, painters like Van Gogh, whose most productive period was the year before his suicide when he was 37, and poets like Byron, Rossetti and Shelley, are known to have experienced periods of intense creative energy punctuated by spells of crippling melancholia, as depression was then known, and it has been suggested that at least some of them suffered from a degree of manic depression apart from their other illnesses.

As with endogenous depression, the cause of manic depression is believed to be a disturbance in brain chemistry, in which heredity is believed to have a key role; but environmental influences also play a part. Evidence of a genetic basis for at least one form of manic depression was provided in 1986 by Dr Janice Egeland of the University of Miami, whose report appeared in the American journal, *Science*. In her research among the Amish people, an isolated religious group which does not allow the use of alcohol or other drugs, Dr Egeland discovered that manic depression within this community was due to a fault affecting a single gene (one of the minute chemical units of heredity which determine an individual's characteristics and, in some cases, vulnerability to certain disorders). In her study of families, she found that only four families were involved in the 26 suicides reported among the group since 1880. (Untreated manic depression has a high suicide risk.)

Doctors have known for a long time that manic depression tends to 'run in families' and that where one family member responds well to drug treatment – usually lithium – other affected members are likely to respond equally well. Dr Egeland's research indicates that, because of a genetic defect, some vital brain chemical which normally has a stabilizing effect on mood is absent from the brain of a susceptible person. This information may provide a clue to the development of future treatment but it should be stressed that not everyone who possesses the faulty gene automatically develops the disorder. In those with a genetic risk, the illness tends to develop usually when triggered by stress and acute anxiety.

An interesting insight into the sufferer's perceptions during the transfer from the depressive to the manic phase was provided by a distinguished British academic at a conference in 1982, who described his own emergence from severe depression (triggered by a serious 'life event'). This occurred after he had listened to a record which was currently on the hit parade: 'It somehow gave me a high and I switched from depression to hypermania. It lasted four months and it was good for me but hell for everyone else.'

About 370,000 people in Britain suffer from manic-depression. In England alone, about 24,000 people with a severe form of the illness are admitted to hospital each year. Correct diagnosis often is delayed because most of those consulting a doctor do so during the depressive phase. The early treatment is likely to be similar to that for reactive depression. Drugs from the tricyclic group of anti-depressants may be given during a depressive phase, followed by a switch to lithium carbonate to treat manic symptoms and prevent further attacks. About three-quarters of patients respond well to lithium therapy (see page 143). For the quarter who do not, other drugs such as carbamazepine (Tegretol) are reported to be helpful.

MASKED DEPRESSION

Also called 'atypical depression', this is thought to be a variant of endogenous depression: the basic problem appears to originate within the sufferer's own mind, and is not necessarily related to some 'life event'. Because the depression is masked and hidden, the sufferer is not aware of feeling depressed apart from complaining about the tiresomeness and discomfort of the masking symptom, usually a long-standing physical complaint of some kind.

The most common chronic symptoms found among patients later diagnosed as having masked depression are: headache, backache, rheumatic pains, poor appetite, indigestion, bowel and bladder irregularities (including diarrhoea and urinary frequency), fatigue, palpitations, dizziness, breathlessness, sleep disturbance, sexual problems and skin complaints (which may be exacerbated by scratching). In such cases, it has been found that the physical symptoms tend to improve rapidly once the illness has been diagnosed correctly and the patient has been given anti-depressant drugs.

That is not to say that the physical complaints are not very real to the patient while they last, of course. All illnesses have some psychosomatic (mind/body) element. The mind can exert a powerful influence over bodily function so that we feel physically ill when we are in fact quite well. And, even in serious illness, our way of thinking about the illness can have a crucial effect on our ability to tolerate the physical and psychological pain which may be associated with it. On the simplest level, we all know that the more we concentrate on a symptom, the worse it seems, which is why a reassuring word from the doctor can make us feel better by allaying anxiety. Acute anxiety, fear and apprehension can bring about temporary biochemical changes in the blood (such as increasing adrenaline to fuel us for the classic 'fight or flight' response) and these can lead to symptoms like dryness of the mouth, dizziness, palpitations, increased pulse rate, raised blood pressure, and urgency with regard to bowel and bladder activity. Who hasn't experienced some of these symptoms before an important exam or a difficult interview!

The patient with masked depression does not always present physical symptoms, however. Behaviour problems can also be an indication, especially where these represent a dramatic change in behaviour. Common pointers are alcoholism, gambling, shoplifting, sexual promiscuity and evidence of increased hostility towards people generally in someone who is normally of an amiable disposition. Because sufferers are less likely to consult the doctor about problems like these, an underlying depression may not be recognized until after a suicide attempt. In elderly people, depression is common, and may be mistaken for signs of dementia, especially where symptoms include impairment of memory and retardation (slowness of movement and speech), which are more readily recognized as evidence of depression in younger people.

Joy was in her early forties by the time she gave up hope of ever finding even a part-time job. 'I suddenly saw myself in a new light, as some sort of middle-aged freak trying to compete with school-leavers and dolly-birds for badly-paid work. After one last round of the agencies I just gave up. I took a last look in the mirror at all the lines and creases I'd never noticed before, and I said, "That's it!" With nothing much to do I got more and more depressed, and the tablets the doctor gave me didn't help a lot after the first few months so I flushed them down the toilet.

'The only thing that seemed to give me a lift was a drink. I started in a small way, just having an occasional glass from the cabinet, but without realizing it I was increasing my intake quite rapidly. Next thing, I was sneaking in gin bottles from the supermarket and hiding the empties until I could sneak them out discreetly to dump somewhere. Alcoholism is a very insidious business. You think you have drink under control until the day you realize you're as completely hooked as if you were on heroin or cocaine. And you can't confide in anyone, least of all your family, because you feel so ashamed. Needless to say, I was soon in debt and that was another problem I wasn't able to handle, though I carried on somehow.

'I suppose it's a fair comment on the plight of women in my position that my family never noticed anything unusual until they came home one evening and I hadn't done anything about preparing a meal. They thought I'd had a stroke or something like it when they found me slumped in an armchair, all groggy and glassy-eyed and talking nonsense. I have no memory of this, but they told me about it later. What I do remember very clearly was my son's expression – so disgusted, so lacking in compassion – when he got a whiff of my breath. "You're drunk!" he said. He kept repeating it until I wanted to scream, but I couldn't produce a sound.

'It was the one thing that got through to me, that look on my son's face. It made me so angry when I thought about it, but it helped in a strange way too. "Start thinking of yourself for a change, my girl," I told myself. "You owe it to yourself to get out of this mess and make something of your life." And somehow I did. It was a hard struggle with a lot of help from Alcoholics Anonymous and another self-help group, but I made it eventually. I don't expect to find paid employment now, but I'm reasonably content doing part-time voluntary work – helping to run a group for people with addiction problems. It's useful work and we all help each other. It's a question of having faith and hope, and taking it one day at a time, as the book says, but I know I daren't have even one drink. As I see it now, I took the easy way out when I was feeling almost suicidal. When you're my age and not used to going out on your own, there is a limit to what you can do by way of self-destructiveness. Getting quietly sloshed in the privacy of your own home is so easy, and this is what happens to a lot of women of all ages.'

For Joy, as for so many others, the 'cure' merely intensified the depression, and brought its own even more intractable problems. Chemically-induced depression due to alcohol abuse is a very common illness; and, to complete the vicious circle, the sort of shattering personal experience which so often leads to depression can also drive people to drink. For the social drinker, alcohol means no more than a pleasant occasion and perhaps a mild hangover. But for someone whose drinking escalates out of control, the after-effects can be devastating. The profound misery and self-loathing which usually accompany withdrawal after a heavy bout of drinking are believed to result from biochemical reaction to dramatic changes in the level of alcohol in the blood. Women are much more vulnerable than men to these and to other damaging effects of alcohol, because of their smaller physical size and metabolic differences (see pages 124-138).

Having become despondent and demoralized in her unsuccessful search for a job, Joy still felt that all would be well if suitable employment were to materialize. She now sees her drift into alcoholism as a desperate attempt to cope with her depression, in much the same way that others take to gambling or shoplifting or abuse of other addictive drugs. Her advice to other women in a similar predicament is: 'Don't wait around hoping for the impossible when your children have grown up. Get out and make new friends – there are lots of things you can do, like taking up a course of study or doing voluntary work. I only wish I had realized this!'

Although doctors are very much aware of the problem of masked depression these days, the condition can be difficult to detect, especially where the patient gives a clear account of the progress of some physical ailment. So it is possible that a patient developing a series of different symptoms over a long period may be referred for the attention of a number of different hospital specialists without any organic basis for these problems being discovered. The final referral – to a psychiatrist – is often the one which provides the answer to the puzzle.

DEPRESSION DUE TO PHYSICAL ILLNESS
One of the many important reasons for seeking medical advice when someone suffers from symptoms of depression is the possibility that the symptoms may be due to a physical condition which requires treatment. It is extremely difficult to feel cheerful when we are aware of bodily pain or discomfort, but at least we know why we are feeling out of sorts. However, there are numerous potentially serious conditions less easily recognized which can give rise to symptoms usually associated with

depression, like apathy, listlessness, tiredness, irritability, lack of energy and loss of interest in customary activities.

In women, one of the most common conditions causing such symptoms is iron-deficiency anaemia associated with the menstrual loss, or with heavier monthly bleeding due to the use of an IUD (intra-uterine contraceptive device). A test to check the level of haemoglobin (the colouring matter of red blood cells) will confirm the existence of this type of anaemia, which can usually be corrected by giving iron supplements. In men and post-menopausal women, iron-deficiency anaemia usually calls for further investigation, on the assumption that there may be some hidden blood loss (such as from a gastric or duodenal ulcer) to account for the problem. There are also other, more complex, forms of anaemia which can cause depressive and physical symptoms in both men and women, for which prompt diagnosis and treatment are essential.

Diabetes mellitus (sugar diabetes) is a condition in which there is a deficiency of insulin, a chemical secreted by the pancreas which regulates sugar metabolism. Depending on its severity, treatment for this deficiency may include insulin injections, other drugs or dietary adjustment. Usually the only obvious early symptoms of untreated diabetes are a very marked increase in thirst and urinary output, which may not be noticed by members of the sufferer's family. Signs which may be noticed are increased irritability, restlessness and depression, weight loss and lowered resistance to infection.

Mood changes and other symptoms of depression can also be due to under- or over-activity of the thyroid gland, a large gland in the front of the neck which stores iodine absorbed in minute quantities from food, and secretes thyroxine, an essential hormone.

The most important function of the thyroid gland is the control of metabolism, the delicate chemical process involved in converting the food we eat into nutrient matter for body tissue, in burning it to provide fuel for energy, and in breaking down waste products for elimination. The thyroid gland works in cooperation with other hormone-producing glands to maintain the body's endocrine balance. (Endocrine or ductless glands produce hormones which pass directly into the bloodstream.) It has an influence on the central nervous system, and on the health of skin and hair; in childhood, it has a crucial impact on physical and mental development.

Under-activity of the thyroid gland (hypothyroidism or myxoedema) produces the symptoms related to its functions listed above. In infancy, deficiency results in a form of delayed development called 'cretinism'. In adults, deficiency can develop so insidiously that patients do not realize they are ill, apart from feelings of lethargy, aches and pains in the joints and general depression. The sufferers – often middle–aged women – tend to gain weight, to have dry skin, dull and falling hair, to be slow in speech, movement and mental functioning, to have a subnormal temperature and a slow pulse rate. Coldness and thickening of the skin and gruffness of the voice are other signs which doctors look for as an indication that the body's metabolic rate has slowed down, when referring a new patient for hospital investigation of thyroid function. In both infancy and adult life, the problem can be treated successfully by giving thyroxine in carefully adjusted doses.

Even when the patient is a doctor, it can happen occasionally that the real source of trouble is overlooked, especially if the symptoms appear to have psychosomatic overtones. The account of her own illness given by a woman physician in *World Medicine* (5 March 1983) certainly provides a salutary lesson. She was aged 24 years when her troubles began.

'I thought I was suffering from a combination of overwork and inadequacy: night work was becoming a problem, and one year later I had to leave the hospital service because I simply could not get up to attend the night calls.'

This marked the beginning of a disturbing and distressing illness which lasted for many years, baffled no fewer than ten teaching hospital consultants and almost convinced her that she was a 'hopeless hypochondriac'. Finally, she was referred to an endocrinologist who diagnosed myxoedema and prescribed thyroxine, the standard replacement treatment which restored her to health. 'I had no idea how well I could feel until I was normal,' she recalled. Now that a blood test is available for the purpose, assessment of thyroid function is a much easier process than in the past.

As may be expected, over-activity of the thyroid gland (hyperthyroidism) has the opposite effects. This is usually associated with the enlargement of the gland known as goitre which, in mild forms, may go unrecognized. Simple goitre arises when the diet lacks iodine (the necessary traces are now found in most drinking water and table salt) and the gland is stimulated to compensate by producing more thyroxine. In the past, this form of goitre was common in mountainous regions of the European continent where the soil lacked iodine, and in England's 'goitre belt' stretching from Derbyshire to Somerset – the term 'Derbyshire neck' was once synonymous with the condition. More complex forms including toxic goitre (thyrotoxicosis, Graves' disease) are believed to be due to malfunction of the thyroid controlling mechanism in the brain rather than to any fault in the gland itself. Treatment can include surgery to reduce thyroid enlargement, drugs to block the effect of excess thyroxine and radioiodine therapy. Neither of these two medical treatments is given during pregnancy because of a possible risk to the foetus.

The majority of sufferers from hyperthyroidism again tend to be middle-aged women. The patient becomes restless and irritable and, while her appetite may often be good, she loses weight, due to an increase in metabolism. Her pulse rate is likely to be rapid, and she may complain of increased sweating and general nervousness. In women of childbearing age, disturbance of menstruation is common. Clinical symptoms may include goitre, exophthalmic signs (protrusion of eyes seen in Graves' disease), and irregularity of the heart-beat. However, a great many sufferers do not have a noticeable degree of thyroid enlargement, which can make the condition more difficult for the doctor to detect in some cases.

A salutary lesson on the ease with which physical

complaints may be mistaken for more serious mental illness – in the United States at least – was provided in a report which appeared in 1979 on a study carried out by Dr Earl Gardner, associate professor of psychiatry at Texas University. When thorough medical tests were conducted among 100 consecutive patients being admitted to a mental hospital, it was discovered that 46 had previously undiagnosed physical ailments which were responsible for their psychiatric symptoms. The patients, whose ages ranged from 18 to 32, included 55 women and 45 men. And 95 per cent of them were being committed on mental health warrants under legal procedure.

The screening process included detailed analysis of blood chemistry and urine, using sophisticated modern equipment available in Britain for upwards of 20 years, together with electro-cardiography and electro-encephalography (respectively to test heart and brain function), and a complete physical examination. The 46 patients found to have physical complaints had between them 186 different conditions affecting health. And 28 of them had disorders of the endocrine glands – glands such as the thyroid which produce vital hormones.

DEPRESSION ASSOCIATED WITH PHYSICAL ILLNESS
This is an understandable reaction, even when the illness is nothing more than a transient bout of influenza. When the illness is more serious, perhaps with life-threatening implications, then anxiety and depression are inescapable. Yet it has been found that, for those facing a major operation or a period in hospital for medical treatment, one of the main causes of fear and apprehension is poor communication between the patient and those providing medical care. Even today, when so much emphasis is being placed on the importance of keeping patients informed, and allowing them a say in the choice of treatment, few patients seem satisfied with the information they are given. *Words* remain one of the scarcest commodities in a National Health Service which continues to function remarkably well despite many vicissitudes.

The tradition of not talking to the patient about anything

as relevant as his illness and treatment dies hard. There certainly are practical and compassionate grounds for not passing on bad news to someone who has not asked to be told the whole truth about a demoralizing prognosis. On the other hand, there is a strong case for offering a clear explanation in terms which the patient can appreciate, when the findings are reassuring. In practice, patients can become unnecessarily despondent when they think that something is being hidden from them. Or, as happened to a friend of mine who was being treated for terminal cancer in a London teaching hospital, they feel betrayed when ticked off by the ward sister for questioning the nurses about their treatment.

Until recently, depression among general hospital patients received relatively little attention, no doubt because providing physical care already placed so many demands on hard-pressed staff. Now that the problem is more widely recognized, it is being found that even severely ill patients are able to respond well to help from a professional counsellor and, where necessary, anti-depressant drugs. With the trend these days towards much earlier discharge from hospital of post-operative patients, the needs of convalescent and chronically ill patients living in their own homes call for special attention from those providing care in the community – GPs, nurses, health visitors, social workers, therapists, clergy and voluntary workers. It is worth remembering that, where the family doctor considers it advisable, certain hospital specialists – such as those in psychiatry and geriatric medicine – can be asked to see patients in their own homes. However, the basic necessity of recognizing that a patient may need treatment for depression often rests with those who are in the best position to notice early tell-tale signs: relatives, home helps and friendly neighbours.

'Psychological disturbances associated with chronic physical illness are based on fear of death or spreading of the disease, incapacity, pain, abandonment and loss of self-esteem,' according to Dr Thomas D. Walsh, research fellow in clinical pharmacology, and Dame Cicely Saunders, medical director in the department of clinical studies, at St Christopher's Hospice, London. Nevertheless they found that despite the universal fear of cancer, severe depression is uncommon among the majority of patients even at an advanced stage, and suicide is rare: 'Patients who are more prone to depression are those who have been misdiagnosed, or deliberately misled, or who have suffered from unsympathetic management.' Others with an increased risk of depression include women (especially those being treated for breast cancer), younger patients, and those with a history of psychological problems. The importance of keeping the patient actively involved in the treatment programme is emphasized, particularly to minimize stress which may be associated with modern cancer treatment, such as cytotoxic drugs and radiotherapy.

'Much harm is done by lying about the diagnosis and prognosis, with irreparable harm to patient-staff-family relationships, and causing many difficulties when the disease progresses.' Even when cure is not possible, the patient and his family should never be left without some hope – for example that distressful 'symptoms will always be relieved'. Very great expertise in the treatment and prevention of severe pain has indeed been developed by staff in the hospice movement, and in the 200 or more NHS pain clinics scattered throughout the country.

Women tend to suffer from depression about breast cancer twice as much as from cancer of any other kind. It is estimated that up to two in every five women having a mastectomy remain depressed and anxious for at least a year afterwards. Problems in sexual relationships are common, largely due to the damage to self-esteem which the loss of a breast can involve, and the woman's fear of rejection if she were to allow her partner to see the resultant scar. Even with the growing practice whereby surgeons try to conserve as much breast tissue as possible, and thus limit disfigurement, a woman may still have to contend with considerable scarring. However, with newer surgical and cosmetic techniques being developed, this should be less of a problem in future.

While it is true that women suffer severe emotional

trauma because of the cosmetic aspects of mastectomy, the health implications of breast cancer, together with the discomfort often associated with additional treatment, are also a source of anxiety and depression. The importance of counselling before and after surgery is widely recognized. Research by a team at the University Hospital of South Manchester has shown that counselling by a specialist nurse can lead to a three-fold reduction in psychological problems associated with mastectomy (*British Medical Journal*, 26 June 1982.

For women who need more intensive psychotherapy to help them to adjust to the loss of a breast, cognitive therapy, with or without anti-depressant drugs, is proving effective in treatment at Prestwich and Hope Hospitals, Manchester, according to a report by Dr Liz Grist (*General Practitioner*, 12 September 1986). With this increasingly popular method, patients are encouraged to alter their way of thinking about a problem, so that they are able to concentrate instead on more positive aspects. She also describes work being done to help male and female cancer sufferers at Gartnavel General Hospital, Glasgow, where psychologists are using progressive muscle relaxation therapy, combined with a lightly induced hypnosis, under which it is suggested that patients would experience a sense of well-being. A study of 71 newly diagnosed patients of both sexes showed a significant reduction in anxiety among those who had been involved in therapy.

Severe depression can be a feature of many other illnesses, including those which have identifiable psychological overtones. An obvious case in point is anorexia nervosa (see pages 105-116). And, as Dr Walsh and Dame Cicely Saunders explain, symptoms of depression may sometimes mislead doctors into missing signs of physical illness. For instance, they say, 'Organic brain disease may produce cognitive impairment, which can be misdiagnosed as due to depression.' On the other hand it is well established that in elderly people, symptoms of treatable depression may be mistaken for untreatable dementia.

DEPRESSION DUE TO DRUGS

Apart from alcohol and drug abuse, which are two major causes of severe depression, a wide range of medicinal drugs can cause depression in some people. Even medication given to treat depression can occasionally aggravate it. The danger of giving benzodiazepine tranquillizers (anti-anxiety drugs) to treat depression was stressed in a 1985 report from Edinburgh, which dealt with the hospital admissions for self-poisoning of 230 adults, of whom the highest proportion were single women aged from 20 to 30 years. These drugs may aggravate existing depression and predispose to suicide, the authors say. Since depression is often accompanied by anxiety, anti-depressant manufacturers are careful to point out which drugs are likely to be most helpful where the two conditions coexist.

It is important, also, to be aware that anti-depressant drugs do not produce immediate relief when a course is begun. Some newer drugs may begin to take effect within a week, but many others may take up to two or three weeks before the full effect is appreciated. Therefore, it should not be assumed that these are of no help or may even be causing depression, or that you would be better off without them (especially if they are causing some temporary but mild side effects). If you are worried, consult your doctor, but don't stop taking the medication unless you are having severe adverse side-effects.

While it is always worth considering whether or not any medicines you are taking may be causing depression, it goes without saying that you should not stop taking an essential medicine on this assumption without your doctor's consent. In fact, some drugs which are known to cause depression in some people may be crucially important to health and well-being, and the doctor may need to consider replacing them with some other treatment. Examples are steroids (for inflammation, allergy and so on); reserpine (for high blood pressure); and the contraceptive pill (in some instances).

In a review in *MIMS Magazine* (Monthly Index of Medical Specialities) in 1984, Dr Alan Lee of the Institute of

Psychiatry in London warned doctors of the need for caution in prescribing these and certain other drugs for patients with a previous history of depression due to any cause. Even a family history of depression should be taken into account, if there is any suspicion of a genetic predisposition. Women and older people have been found to be physiologically more susceptible to drug-induced depression but, while over 250 prescribed drugs have been mentioned by doctors at various times as a possible cause of depression, only a small number have actually been shown to have this effect, Dr Lee explained. It is always advisable when seeing the doctor because of depression or anxiety —·or indeed for any other reason – to mention all medicines being taken, including those purchased from the chemist, and herbal remedies.

Interaction between different drugs can also cause depression and other problems. One of the most common and dangerous types of interaction is that which can occur when alcohol is combined with drugs of abuse like heroin, or prescribed drugs such as anti-depressants and tranquillizers, since all of these have a depressant effect on vital biochemical activity in the brain. And, because women's bodies are less efficient than men's bodies in coping with alcohol, they are much more likely to suffer severe depression during the withdrawal phase after a drinking bout. For both sexes, there is a serious risk to life in combining alcohol and other drugs, through loss of consciousness and asphyxiation owing to inhalation of vomited material.

Some drugs cause depression when they are withdrawn. This can be one of the withdrawal symptoms of tranquillizers, which should always be stopped gradually by reducing the dosage over a period of time. Stimulant drugs like amphetamines, and some appetite suppressants used to treat obesity (which act on the central nervous system), can also cause depression if stopped suddenly. Manufacturers advise doctors to be particularly cautious in prescribing many of these anti-obesity drugs for patients prone to depression; and they should not be given to anyone already taking MAOI anti-depressants.

DEPRESSION AND OTHER HEALTH PROBLEMS IN OLD AGE

Depression is believed to be very common among elderly people. Yet it tends to be under-diagnosed or mistaken for dementia. One reason for this is that the sufferer seldom complains of feeling depressed. Another is that many symptoms of severe depression are similar to those also seen in dementia, such as apathy, loss of interest in surroundings, slowness in movement, speech and response to questions, and memory impairment. Elderly people are also much more prone to depression and mental confusion associated with drug treatment. Because they tend to suffer from an increasing number of physical ailments, they often have a variety of drugs prescribed, which they may or may not take in strict accordance with medical instructions. Indeed, studies have shown that quite a high proportion of hospital admissions among the very elderly are for illnesses which are due directly to adverse effects of prescribed drugs.

It is not unusual for such medicines to be supplied on a 'repeat prescription' basis, without the doctor seeing the patient each time the supply of drugs is renewed. Perhaps because they do not always remember the instructions given when their medicines were first prescribed, and because they don't know enough about them to recognize adverse reaction, elderly people may not even think of attributing additional physical or psychological symptoms to the drugs they are taking. Yet it is well known that as we grow older, our bodies are less well able to deal efficiently with drugs than when we were younger.

Sometimes symptoms such as dizziness and 'funny turns', which can be very frightening, are due to sudden movement or to the effects of drugs. Dizziness which occurs on rising in the morning or when getting out of a warm bath is often due to 'postural hypotension', which means that there is a temporary drop in the blood supply to the brain. This can occur at any age, but it is more common in elderly people, who are bound to feel anxious and to lose self-confidence if they don't understand how it happens and don't realize that it can often be avoided by modifying regular routine: by first rising into a sitting position and resting for a time before getting out of bed, for instance.

'When an adult stands, 500ml of blood is pooled in the legs and simply lost to the circulation,' Professor Michael Lye of the Royal Liverpool Hospital, explained in an article on the subject (*Pulse*, 20 October 1984). In infancy, our bodies learn how to bring special postural reflexes into action to compensate for this temporary deficiency. But with ageing these reflexes tend to become less efficient, and so we are more prone to dizziness produced by a sudden lowering of blood pressure when we stand up suddenly.

Many drugs can also cause these postural reflexes to work less efficiently, and these include drugs commonly prescribed for elderly people to treat high blood pressure, or irregularities of the heart rhythm, or psychological problems such as anxiety or depression. Professor Lye's list includes, in addition to diuretics (drugs to increase urinary output) and other drugs to treat high blood-pressure – tricyclic and MAOI anti-depressants; antihistamines (in common cold cures, travel sickness pills and pills for allergic conditions); minor tranquillizers (for anxiety); and major tranquillizers (used in treatment of psychotic illness). He also includes barbiturates, frequently used in the past to treat depression and insomnia, but now on the restricted drugs list because of the risks they involve, and says that where symptoms of postural hypotension are thought to be due to any of these drugs, the solution may be for the doctor to reduce dosage, or to start with low doses and increase dosage very gradually.

Digoxin – often combined with a diuretic – is a drug commonly prescribed to correct irregularities of heart rhythm in elderly people. It has the effect of slowing and strengthening the heart-beat and pulse-rate and is, therefore, a very valuable drug which needs to be taken strictly according to instructions. On the other hand, digoxin can sometimes cause depression, especially when it is combined with a diuretic. It can occasionally have a cumulative effect in the body which, if recognized, may prompt the doctor to reduce the daily dosage temporarily.

If patients or their relatives learn to check the pulse in the wrist, they can recognize abnormal slowing – below 60 beats a minute – which might indicate that the digoxin dosage is too high, and they should telephone the doctor for advice. At the same time, it is important not to get into the habit of checking the pulse-rate unnecessarily when one feels perfectly well, as this can lead to needless worry and anxiety.

Both depression and one form of dementia can be treated successfully in elderly people. Dementia is a condition in which there usually is loss of memory, personality changes, failure of intellectual powers, and inability to carry out many of the ordinary tasks involved in daily living. It is estimated that about three-quarters of a million elderly people in Britain suffer from this condition, that is, six per cent of the elderly population, and the highest proportion of these are among the over-80 age-group. Four-fifths of patients live in their own homes, where support for the family may be provided by the GP, a home help, visiting community psychiatric and general nurses, social workers and, where possible, attendance at a psychogeriatric day hospital.

Dementia is broadly divided into reversible and irreversible confusional states, according to their causes. The reversible forms develop rapidly in response to disruption of brain function brought about by injury or disease (stroke or brain tumour, for instance); by very high fever associated with infectious disease; by toxic substances from infections or diseases such as liver or kidney failure; by alcohol or drug overdose; and by certain severe nutritional deficiencies. Irreversible dementia develops more gradually, and is due to degeneration and loss of brain cells essential for the efficient use of speech, memory and movement skills. The most common form of this in the elderly is called Alzheimer's disease.

Something like 95 per cent of elderly people live in their own homes. Depression among them is said to be on the increase, due to loneliness, isolation, impaired mobility and other disabling conditions, material hardship and chronic ill-health. One of the saddest of the many sad

47

developments reported in 1986 was the news of a steep rise in attempted suicide among elderly people (*Pulse*, 20–27 December 1986). A survey reported by Dr John Merrill, psychiatrist with the West Midlands Poisons Unit, showed that deliberate self-poisoning rates among those aged 65 and over had more than doubled in the last two years, with women predominant among the casualties. A high incidence of depression and physical illness was reported among the group studied and, in the majority of cases, self-poisoning was judged to be a serious suicide attempt.

As a nation, we don't worry very much about the comfort, well-being or quality of life of our elderly citizens, which is why Age Concern found it necessary to launch a national campaign for 1987 on the theme 'Celebrating Age'. The aim of the campaign was to highlight positive aspects of older age, and the valuable contribution which older people can make to our society. Let us hope that this worthy cause wins the success it deserves, and which elderly people so badly need in the late 1980s.

Finally, we must not forget the personal welfare needs of relatives who care for the majority of mentally and physically frail elderly people – whose own well-being has been virtually ignored over the years, apart from the pioneering efforts of a few voluntary organizations.

It requires no great feat of imagination to realize that caring for a mentally frail elderly person is a daunting and depressing responsibility, from which there is little respite. We tend to assume that, because support services (and in some cases an invalid care allowance) are now available through the NHS and DHSS, local authority social services and voluntary organizations, everyone who needs this help is receiving it. In fact, this assumption is often far from the truth. The invalid care allowance is not available to women over 60 who form a large proportion of carers. Writing in the nursing journal *Community View* (July 1986), Judith Oliver, director of the Association of Carers, reported on her association's research:

'Nearly 70 per cent of carers are, at any one time, injured or ill. So we are not looking at able-bodied young people taking care of the frail or handicapped . . . An elderly member caring for her mother who was in her nineties had, eventually, to find £380 for a place in a private nursing home in order that she herself could go and have a hip replacement. Though all the statutory agencies with whom she was in touch were fully aware of her needs, her mother was rejected for a hospital bed for the duration ("She isn't actually ill") and rejected by the local authority for a bed in an old people's home ("She's too confused and incontinent for our staff to cope with").'

On the question of home-visiting health care professionals, Ms Oliver found that many community nurses truly believed that every severely disabled person in their area was known to them and receiving their help. 'Far from it. The majority of carers and patients never see a nurse,' she says. In fairness, it should be added that communication within the statutory services is by no means perfect in all areas. Liaison between family doctors and the social services department often is extremely poor, especially where the GP's practice cannot call on the help of an attached nurse or social worker. Moreover, community nurses usually take on new patients through direct referral from the patient's GP. If a carer seems to be managing quite well, and if the patient does not require regular treatment such as an injection or dressings for pressure sores or leg ulcers, the doctor may not consider it necessary for a nurse to call unless this service is requested.

SEASONAL AFFECTIVE DISORDER (SAD)
In younger people this is a relatively rare form of depression which is believed to be directly related to a sharp decrease during the darker days of winter and early spring in the amount of daylight entering the eyes and reaching the brain via the optic nerves. Understood to be similar in nature to endogenous and manic-depression, SAD sets in each autumn and lifts automatically with the return of late spring and summer sunlight.

The majority of those susceptible tend to be women and older people, who find that they sleep more, consume more carbohydrate foods, put on weight and become increasingly lethargic as autumn fades into winter.

49

The explanation put forward by the numerous scientists who have studied this phenomenon is that changes in light levels may cause an imbalance in the levels of the sleep-inducing brain chemical, melatonin. Normally, melatonin production increases at night and decreases in the early morning in response to light messages transmitted via the optic nerves to the pineal gland in the brain. Where someone is susceptible to SAD, the theory is that the dull daylight of late autumn, winter and early spring is not enough to operate the chemical switch, and so melatonin levels remain abnormally high throughout the day, causing lethargy, weariness and dejection of spirits.

The existence of seasonal variations in depression among elderly people has been recognized for many years. One of the first psychogeriatricians to study the problem was Dr Colin Godber of Moorgreen Hospital, Southampton. He observed among his elderly patients a marked increase in the incidence of depression and suicide, which reached a peak in early summer and the pre-Christmas period and which was probably related to rapid alterations in daylight hours up to two or three months earlier. Because of their general frailty, elderly people prone to biological (endogenous) depression may be particularly susceptible to SAD, owing to a drop in the efficiency of regulating brain chemistry.

One of the most comprehensive studies into seasonal depression in general was conducted by Dr Alec Coppen, who has carried out neuropsychiatry laboratory research on behalf of the Medical Research Council in Britain and the World Health Organization. In a month-by-month assessment of variations in the body's biochemistry, he discovered very marked fluctuations – varying by as much as 30 per cent throughout the year – in the levels of another brain chemical, serotonin, which tend to be reduced in endogenous depression (*Pulse*, 26 January 1985). Conversely, it is suggested that excessively high levels of serotonin may be the triggering factor for an attack of schizophrenia in some sufferers prone to this disorder.

It is to be hoped that SAD, like other disorders due to an imbalance in brain chemistry, can be treated one day by medication designed to restore equilibrium. Considerable research is being directed towards this goal. In the meantime, sufferers are being helped by conventional treatment, including anti-depressant drugs and, where necessary, electroconvulsive therapy (ECT). But for a growing number of patients and their doctors, the use of special lighting to treat seasonal affective disorder represents a novel and potentially viable alternative to older methods. Studies to evaluate the technique are being carried out at British hospitals, such as Charing Cross and Maudsley Hospitals in London, where encouraging results have been reported.

A suggestion that children may sometimes be prone to SAD was made in a report published in 1986 in the *American Journal of Psychiatry*. It advises that the disorder should be considered as a possibility in children who develop problems during winter, such as fatigue, irritability, sleep disturbances and difficulties at school. The report describes the cases of seven children believed to be suffering from SAD. Their symptoms improved dramatically after a course of artificial daylight treatment or 'phototherapy', which is widely used for the treatment of SAD in the United States.

The pioneer who developed phototherapy for SAD is Dr Norman Rosenthal of the National Institute of Mental Health in Maryland. In his own studies he found that depressed patients experienced a dramatic improvement in mood when exposed to strong lighting equivalent to that of a bright spring day; and that they suffered a relapse if the treatment was abandoned. Therapeutic 'exposure' involved being awake so that light could enter the eyes but not necessarily remaining idle in the presence of the light for a period of three hours, morning and evening. So far, medical use of the technique has been limited in Britain, although suppliers of the necessary equipment say there is an increasing trend towards self-treatment. However, they warn against attempting phototherapy without consulting a doctor. No matter how simple the concept seems, this is a physical treatment aimed at bringing about changes in brain chemistry and, therefore, the individual's problems and existing treatment need to be taken into account.

CHAPTER 3

Slaves of our hormones?

Ironically, at a time when women are striving for recognition as competent and responsible workers in their own right at all levels in their chosen fields, there still exists a school of thought which – albeit unintentionally – does much to perpetuate the myth of feminine frailty. The widespread publicity focused recently on problems associated with the menstrual cycle is hardly likely to have enhanced the promotional prospects of women, or boosted their morale. What Victorian feminists called 'this monstrous cult of female invalidism' is still alive and flourishing in the 1980s. Prominent physicians may no longer murmur discreetly about the ills of 'a lady's poorly times' or 'monthly returns' – or insist that 'consumption is produced by failure of the menstrual function', but some still make seemingly inordinate claims for premenstrual tension and the menopause as major causes of depression and more serious psychiatric disorders among women. 'Are your hormones giving you trouble again?' a cheeky subordinate asked his woman boss in an American film shown on British television not long ago. The scriptwriter was a man, needless to say.

In the childbearing years, premenstrual tension is regarded as the great bogey which can, at worst, turn a healthy woman into a semi-invalid, a dangerous driver, a petty criminal or potentially violent individual for several days in the month. There have even been instances where a history of very severe premenstrual disorder has been accepted by the criminal courts as a mitigating factor in serious offences. No doubt, there are many women who suffer great distress for which specialist care is needed, but is the problem as prevalent as some authorities seem to claim? Surely the experience of those of us who have worked with large numbers of women, in jobs like hospital nursing, suggests that it is not.

And what about the alleged terrors of the menopause, which previous generations of women are said to have welcomed as a release from the risk of repeated pregnancies? Is this event usually accompanied by as much physical and emotional discomfort as we have been led to expect? Hardly, though here too there are exceptions, cases of women who do need hormone supplements to alleviate unusually severe or persistent symptoms commonly associated with the menopause. However, it is fair to assume that much of the dread surrounding the menopause stems from the sort of conditioning which leads women to accept the end of their childbearing potential as virtually the end of life too.

No doubt the fact that most severe forms of depression tend to affect women during the childbearing years has lent weight to the view that hormonal changes are likely to be responsible in many cases. This opinion is no longer shared by all contemporary authorities, however. With better understanding of the role of social factors in emotional disorders, it is being recognized that the childbearing years are also the years when the general stresses of life tend to weigh most heavily on us all. In a comprehensive review of research on the subject, psychology lecturer Doreen Asso concluded that premenstrual depression, when it occurs, tends to be short-lived and has few of the features associated with clinical depression.

Medical perceptions of the menopause have also changed radically in recent years. No longer is this regarded as a potential catastrophe affecting large numbers of women for whom oestrogen therapy ('hormone replacement therapy') is an essential treatment. The current situation was summed up in a recent *British Medical Journal* article by Professor Anthony Clare of St Bartholomew's Hospital, London, and Dr Rachel Jenkins. Their view is that while hormone fluctuations can affect mood, the bulk of medical and sociological evidence indicates an environmental rather than a biological basis for higher rates of depression in women throughout their lives. 'A decade ago it was argued that upwards of 40 per cent of women suffer from post-menopausal syndrome. Today's estimate is 10 per cent and falling,' they say.

Recent research carried out by Professor Martin Vessey and his team in Oxford also confirms earlier British and American studies which found that the menopause does not in itself cause psychiatric problems. While some women may have symptoms which benefit from oestrogen supplements, it is claimed that giving oestrogen has little effect in counteracting depression which coincides with the menopause.

It has often been noted that fashions in illness and treatment tend to vary according to the level of public interest involved. It is also true that reports of serious research often tend to be exaggerated or misunderstood in popular press accounts of a 'breakthrough' or 'scare story' relating to health. So it is not really so surprising that few of today's doctors are as enthusiastic about the virtues of oestrogen therapy as some were during the great 'hype' in its favour some years ago. No doubt disenchanted to discover that synthetic oestrogens do not really hold the key to perpetual youth, and may have unwelcome side-effects, women themselves are now slower to ask their doctors for this treatment. An obvious lesson to be learnt from this episode of medical history is that you should seek treatment only if you feel you really need it. Avoid medicines you don't need – they are unlikely to do you much good, and may even do some harm.

POST-NATAL DEPRESSION
One form of illness in which hormones are believed to have a major role, although social and personal factors have a place too, is post-natal depression. Most mothers experience transient 'blues' and weepiness at some time during the first week after a baby is born but, while hormone changes may partly cause this, there are usually other explanations for their depression. For one thing, there is a sense of anti-climax when the mother may well feel tired and neglected following a period of intense activity and high drama when she was the recipient of so

much attention. Then there is her understandable anxiety about coping with a new baby in her own home, especially if it is her first baby, and she feels nervous about her own capabilities.

Fortunately, most mothers suffering from post-natal illness are able to stay in their own homes. Obviously, the cooperation of husbands and other close relatives is very important, but further care can be provided by GPs, community psychiatric nurses, social workers and health visitors, according to the woman's needs. In many areas, valuable help may be obtained from a local branch of the National Childbirth Trust.

Post-natal illness severe enough to need special hospital treatment is rare. Rarer still is the severest form, post-natal psychosis, which affects one or two new mothers per thousand, and tends to occur between a fortnight and three months after childbirth. If the mother experiences schizophrenia-type symptoms, such as temporary disturbance of thought processes, hearing imaginary voices and so on, it may be considered advisable to admit her and her baby to a special hospital unit. As in all cases of mental disorder, marital and family discord is believed to have an aggravating effect on this illness. But suggestions that modern 'high-tech' intervention in labour may be an important contributory factor have been discounted, on the grounds that the incidence of post-natal psychosis has not increased noticeably over many years.

It is thought that something more than the normal hormone switch from pregnancy to post-natal levels must be present to trigger severe post-natal illness in a small proportion of mothers. One theory is that some malfunction of the thyroid gland may be involved; another is that powerful lactation hormones, stimulating the milk flow for breast-feeding, may sometimes cause disturbance of brain chemistry.

The average hospital stay for post-natal psychosis is six weeks, with treatment which may include anti-depressant drugs, psychotherapy and sometimes ECT (electro-convulsive therapy).

CHAPTER 4

Neurotic illnesses

In everyday life the term 'neurotic' is a label we tend to apply tolerantly to people whose behaviour we regard as being in some way strange, unusual or eccentric: the 'hypochondriac' friend whose health is a constant preoccupation; the over-conscientious colleague who worries unnecessarily; the sensitive relative who is forever taking offence where none is intended. Usually, the only real difference between us and them is that they feel free to express their anxieties and fears more openly than we can – and they may be all the better for it.

In the medical sense, neurotic illness is a disorder which occurs when the sadnesses, worries and fears common to everyone get out of hand and interfere with our enjoyment of life. Unlike a psychotic illness, a neurosis does not affect mental clarity or our understanding of events. What neurotic illness can do, if untreated, is to disrupt our lives very substantially because while we are totally absorbed with our own problems, we have difficulty in concentrating on other matters.

Neurotic illness is the most common type of mental disorder. Fortunately, it can usually be treated successfully by means of counselling, prescribed medication and, where necessary, psychotherapy. Neuroses tend to be classified according to the symptom which appears to be causing most trouble for the sufferer, but all categories have many features in common. For example, anxiety and depression tend to be symptoms of all forms of neurosis, whatever the predominant problem, whereas over-breathing (hyperventilation; see pages 70-73) is a practice usually associated with acute anxiety, panic and phobic attacks.

It used to be thought that neurotic illness was 'all in the

mind', something for which we ourselves or others close to us were responsible. While there is still no doubt that relationships and personal circumstances play a large part, research suggests that the starting point for neurotic illness may be some minute deviation in brain chemistry, just as disorders like endogenous depression and schizophrenia are now seen as essentially physical in their origin.

Newer techniques, such as tomography 'brain scans', and the information thus revealed, have revolutionized specialists' understanding of brain chemistry, and of the precise functions of different areas of the brain in relation to factors such as mood and memory. In a symposium (*Psychiatry in Practice*, May 1985), Dr Michael Trimble of the National Hospital for Nervous Diseases, London, spoke of the 'neurology of the emotions', and advances in knowledge likely to lead to more effective treatment for emotional problems in the foreseeable future. For instance, certain abnormalities of metabolism (chemical changes involved in food processing within the body) have been identified in the brain chemistry of sufferers from panic disorder. Another important step forward was the discovery of neuro-transmitter (chemical messenger) receptors for benzodiazepines (drugs used to treat anxiety) located in the temporal lobe, the area of the brain extending laterally on either side from behind the ear to the temple.

The following conditions come into the category of neuroses:

Anxiety – in an acute form this is the most frequent manifestation of neurotic illness.

Panic attacks – a condition closely allied to anxiety in which sudden, overwhelming fear and physical symptoms are the predominant features.

Phobic anxiety – incapacitating neurosis in which the main symptom is sustained irrational fear of some object or situation.

Obsessive-compulsive disorder – a rarer condition involving increasing preoccupation with a specific idea, and a compulsion to carry out certain rituals related to it, for example, morbid fear of 'germ' contamination and compulsive hand-washing.

Hysteria – the precipitating factor in some cases of chronic physical illness or in loss of function for which no physical cause can be found, for example, temporary blindness or paralysis.

Personality disorder – not a clinical illness but an 'umbrella' category which includes a wide variety of 'deviant' attitudes and behaviour, at a level where they interfere with an individual's social adjustment, possibly including some forms of addiction and criminal behaviour.

ANXIETY

In milder forms, which are in no way related to neurotic illness, anxiety is always with us. It is the vital force which keeps us on the alert for any threat to our own survival or to the well-being of those in our care, and as such it is a normal part of our psychological make-up, a highly efficient early-warning system which keeps us on our guard against physical hazards, reminds us to pay fuel bills and gets us to work on time. Even when it outstrips the bounds of everyday experience, and we are literally 'sick with worry' over family illness or some other crisis, anxiety remains a perfectly normal response which we understand and can usually take in our stride. Occasionally, however, the pressures of life become too great or too numerous for us to deal with, and this is the point at which normal anxiety may persist to a degree in which we experience the sort of symptoms which doctors attribute to neurotic illness. Such neurotic anxiety can occur at any age. It is believed to affect about five per cent of the adult population, of whom women are the majority.

Anxiety and depression are so closely linked that up to 80 per cent of sufferers from anxiety are found to be depressed and vice versa. Because these conditions may call for different approaches to treatment, it is important for the doctor to discover whether anxiety or depression is the predominant problem when someone needs help. One major difference is that depression tends to be triggered off by something which has already happened, whereas anxiety is characterized by acute fear and apprehension concerning some future threat.

In theory, then, anxiety should be one of the easiest symptoms for doctors to detect. In practice, however, allowance has to be made for the sort of everyday nervousness most patients experience when entering the doctor's surgery for a consultation. Watch-checking, foot-shuffling, handkerchief-twisting and the occasional giggle are ploys in which most of us engage at awkward moments. The fact is that it takes considerable courage to walk into the doctor's surgery and say simply, 'My problem is that I feel very anxious most of the time these days.' Even when you know that this is what is disturbing your sleep, affecting your appetite and making you feel permanently tired, the words do not seem to add up to a good enough reason for 'wasting the doctor's time', or so you tell yourself.

So the doctor has to play guessing games – if he can spare the time. Perhaps he will arrive at the correct diagnosis by asking the right questions and observing telling non-verbal signals, such as a patient's refusal to meet his gaze: denial of eye contact is a 'very powerful message of avoidance', we are told. But what a waste of time! How helpful it would be if, instead of being coy and elusive in communication, patients were actively encouraged to speak out confidently and straightforwardly about their emotions, as well as about their physical complaints.

From the sufferer's view-point, neurotic anxiety usually means being permanently 'on edge' over a protracted period without being able to point to a single cause for worry. Very often, however, an attack occurs some time after a person has been under considerable strain concerning problems which had eventually been resolved, as Janet explains:

'It had been a terrible year for illness and trouble in the family. My husband was made redundant and started drinking heavily for the first time in his life. My mother died after a long illness, during which I looked after her. My teenage son and daughter were going off the rails in different ways, and I was convinced that the boy was dabbling in drugs. My sister's marriage broke up, and she spent some time in hospital with nervous trouble. To make matters worse, we were getting into serious financial difficulties, and it looked as if we weren't going to be able to keep up our mortgage payments, and we would soon be homeless. My husband and I quarrelled all the time about his drinking – incidentally, he never stopped until he had frittered away the last penny of his redundancy money. The only thing that kept me sane was my job in the accounts department of a large store, where I had to forget about my personal problems during working hours.

'Then, gradually, things began to get sorted out. My husband found another job and stopped drinking. My son and daughter found new interests and seemed to settle down. My sister seemed to be getting over her depression and was making new friends. But for a long time I would wake up in the morning worrying about them all. Even when I began to feel more relaxed, I would keep reminding myself how awful the nightmare had been; and then I would cross my fingers and convince myself that I mustn't stop worrying! I had got it into my head somehow that misfortunes never happened so long as you were on guard against them – that they were lying in wait to take you by surprise as soon as you relaxed. It's a very illogical way of thinking, but at the time it seemed to work. After about six months, I finally began to believe that everything was going to be all right, and that I could afford to relax my control a bit. And this was the point where *I* began to fall apart.

'It started with the occasional dizzy spell and feeling for a moment as if I couldn't breathe. Then I was having pains in my chest, and palpitations as if my heart was running out of control. The dizzy spells began getting worse, and always seemed to be happening at the most awkward times, especially when I was in the middle of a group of people.

'This was the beginning of a long spell of ill-health which lasted for nearly five years and made my life a misery. I developed urinary problems and chronic diarrhoea and stomach trouble and I couldn't sleep, and at least once a year I saw a different hospital specialist. And no-one seemed to know why I was having dizzy spells, which persisted throughout the illness. It didn't help that I had to change my doctor a couple of times – once when my old GP retired and again when we moved house. It was only when a new GP joined the practice and read the bulging notes in my file that my problems got sorted out finally. After I had gone over my medical history with him, he surprised me by saying that, according to the numerous investigations I'd had, I seemed to be pretty healthy basically. What he reckoned was wrong was that I had been suffering from untreated anxiety all the time, and that it was time to try a different approach. He explained how the anxiety might be causing the physical problems, and how in turn each new symptom gave a fresh boost to the anxiety, creating a vicious circle.

'It was the first time that anyone had mentioned the word 'anxiety' to me – in fact it was the first time I had received an explanation that I could understand. I was given tranquillizers, which I continued taking for three months, and I saw a community psychiatric nurse for counselling once a week, which I also found very helpful. It was like a new lease of life, and I've never looked back really, although I realize that it could happen again if I'm not careful'.

Janet's reference to her bulging medical file describes a phenomenon known to doctors as 'fat file syndrome', which applies to patients who turn up frequently with physical complaints for which no organic cause can be found. The official label for this condition is Briquet's syndrome, so-called after the French doctor who described it in the course of a treatise on hysteria in 1859. Women are not alone in their tendency to translate emotional difficulties into puzzling manifestations of physical illness, of course. Men too have their problems, although very few of them are taken over by anxiety and stress to the extremes reported by Dr Michael O'Donnell in his recent account of a 'pregnant grandfather' (*Guardian*, 14 January 1987), who became a television personality for a day when he was 79 years old and in the throes of his thirtieth pregnancy. This sufferer from the condition known as 'couvade syndrome' experienced problems only when his daughters and grand-daughters were having their babies. With each of their pregnancies his abdomen became swollen and remained so until the baby was born. So far, none of the textbooks has been able to explain what actually goes on in the man's belly on these occasions, according to Dr O'Donnell. Clearly, this is a more distressing experience than the couvade *practised* in some primitive societies, where the tradition is for fathers to lie-in while mothers deliver the babies without fuss and then carry on working in the fields.

Symptoms of anxiety
Symptoms of anxiety include both psychological and physical problems of varying severity. Not everyone experiences all the symptoms at the same time, nor is the sufferer always aware that physical problems are in any way related to anxiety, whereas urinary frequency or persistent diarrhoea are in fact its common accompaniments. Two other conditions which doctors think may often be due to anxiety are recurrent 'cystitis' (inflammation of the bladder and urinary outlet) of the non-infective type which troubles many women, and 'irritable bowel syndrome' (characterized by frequent loose motions, flatulence and abdominal pain). Obviously, such problems need to be investigated to discover whether they really are due to some physical ailment which requires treatment. It is also worth remembering that too much strong coffee or even strong tea can produce nervous symptoms.

The symptoms of anxiety which tend to worry us most and send us in search of medical reassurance are, however, predominantly physical. This is because acute anxiety sets in motion certain changes in body chemistry which are related to the 'fight or flight' instinct – the evolutionary mechanism designed to protect us from imminent danger and to enable us to cope with a crisis.

In moments of stress, a potent chemical called adrenaline is released into the bloodstream by the suprarenal glands, two small bodies sited above each kidney. Through the action of adrenaline, and that of a related substance called noradrenaline, mental and muscle power is placed on the alert to deal with the threatening situation. This is a normal process widely acknowledged in our everyday conversation, of course. We are all familiar with the 'chat show' personality who, when questioned about some spectacular achievement, says modestly: 'I really didn't know how I was going to face it. Then, suddenly, I could feel the adrenaline flowing, and I knew I was going to be all right.' Feeling 'the adrenaline flowing' is the sort of 'high' we need in times of crisis, but it is not a pleasant sensation to have to live with on a long-term basis, as can happen under stress. And, as we all know, too much stress can predispose us to some serious illnesses, including heart disease.

The most noticeable effect adrenaline can have in the body is a series of dramatic changes such as palpitations, increased heart-beat, raised blood-pressure, muscle tension, sweating, and dryness of the mouth. Think of that heart-stopping sense of shock you get on suddenly hearing bad news, or when you feel frightened for some reason or, to a lesser extent, when someone says something which makes you very angry. One way in which your body responds to the situation is to make you feel tense and shaken for some time afterwards. One of adrenaline's main effects is to constrict the arteries, so that blood-pressure and heart-beat are increased, and the circulation to the brain and muscles is stepped up in readiness for action. As part of this diversionary process, there is a temporary decrease in the blood supply to the small peripheral blood vessels underneath the skin, resulting in the pallor we associate with severe stress. The liver is stimulated to act, so that additional glucose from its sugar store is released into the bloodstream to provide extra energy for the muscles. Adrenaline relaxes the muscles of the air passages to stimulate breathing and increase oxygen intake, encourages sweating to keep the body cool, and reduces the secretion of saliva, resulting in a dry mouth.

Diagnosing anxiety
Because of the many similarities in the psychological effects of anxiety and depression, and the physical symptoms for which help is sought, doctors have worked out various methods which help them to distinguish between the two

conditions. Recognition of key clues to anxiety has enabled doctors to structure their questioning of the patient in the best way to elicit information about feelings as distinct from physical problems, which may be crucial to diagnosis.

The results of a survey among women sufferers from anxiety, reported by Professor Robert Priest of St Mary's Hospital, Paddington, shows the rate at which they experienced five different physical symptoms common to anxiety: 73 per cent of the women complained of palpitations and breathlessness; 68 per cent had difficulty in getting to sleep; 60 per cent had trouble with their hands shaking; 47 per cent found that they sweated easily; 43 per cent complained of tension pain in the neck. (Neck and shoulder pains and recurrent tension headache are symptoms more often associated with anxiety than the sufferer may suspect.)

Key questions to which an affirmative answer indicates anxiety are included in The Anxiety and Depression Scale, a 68-item questionnaire described by Professor Donald Eccleston of the Royal Victoria Infirmary, Newcastle-upon-Tyne (*MIMS Magazine*, 1 February 1984). Severely anxious patients are more likely to say 'yes' when asked the following questions:

- Do you feel you often can't get your breath?
- Do you often feel your pulse racing?
- Do you often have palpitations?
- Do you feel panicky in a crowd?
- Do you often feel giddy or faint?
- Are you, or would you be, frightened of travelling on a bus?

Trials have shown that patients with anxiety neurosis are differentiated from those with reactive depression by these six items in the questionnaire, and from those with endogenous depression if they answer 'yes' to a further three questions:

- Do you often nervously perspire or sweat?
- Do you often feel nervous and shaky?
- Do you get a lot of headaches?

Not everyone suffering from anxiety experiences all of these symptoms, of course. But knowing that, more often than not, a combination of them is likely to point to anxiety rather than to some physical problem can be reassuring for the sufferer, says Margaret, a hospital psychotherapist:

'In the average general practice catchment area, there are likely to be hundreds of people walking about who are convinced they are seriously ill because of symptoms like these. In my work I meet people – predominantly women – who have more or less given up work and confined themselves to the house because of symptoms like palpitations and dizzy spells, which they see as a justification for invalidism and perhaps a threat to life. Yet once they have had a reassuring explanation from a doctor they can begin to make an adjustment. However, it doesn't help at all if they are left with the idea that they imagined their physical complaints, because this can make them feel foolish. Sometimes it can take time to help patients to understand that their symptoms were truly physical, and how they came about. For this reason, many need extra support, sometimes ranging from simple counselling to more intensive psychotherapy.'

PANIC ATTACKS

'You never forget your first panic attack,' says Kate, a nurse and mother of two grown-up sons, who is in her mid-forties. She had her first and only full-blown panic attack ten years ago, but the 'fear of fear' remains with her.

'It was the most frightening experience of my life, and I don't think that anyone who has not had an attack can imagine what it is like. I *knew* I was dying, and that it was actually happening at that moment. But because I have survived the ordeal, I don't think I could ever be so terrified again. Nevertheless, I try not to take any chances. Once I'd had the condition explained to me, I developed a strategy for fighting off further attacks when I thought I felt myself about to be taken over. I've been very lucky so far.

'I think the best way to explain it is that some sort of force seems to take you over physically, without warning. I can remember my own panic attack very clearly. I was watching television one Sunday evening and feeling quite relaxed. Then, suddenly, I felt as if I was literally disintegrating. My eyes stopped focusing, so that the picture on the television screen was just a jumble of fuzzy lines. I felt dizzy and I couldn't breathe. My mouth was dry. I had a tight feeling in my chest and I got the impression that my heart was racing. I felt myself going hot and cold in turns. I was shaking all over but I had no feeling in my hands or feet. I was aware of perspiration dripping from my forehead, which I put down to weakness. I believed that I was having a heart attack or a stroke, or maybe a combination of both.

'I remember thinking that I couldn't just sit there and die without doing anything about it. I was surprised to find that I could stand up and walk to the door of the room, although I had great difficulty in breathing. The doctor must be called, I realized: even if he couldn't do much to help, he would be able to give me a sedative. I called my husband, who was doing something in another room, and asked him to telephone and say it was a case of emergency. He became very anxious and concerned, which made me even more agitated, so I commanded him to go and sit down while I prepared for bed. I seemed to be moving about in a trance, unable to breathe, but still managing to tidy up the bedroom for the doctor's visit. It didn't even occur to me that this was extraordinary behaviour, considering that I thought I was dying!

'The doctor came very soon, and I gave him a description of my symptoms quite clearly – I think – although I felt so ill. I remember stressing the fact that I couldn't breathe, and that several times he said, "But you *are* breathing and you are going to go on breathing." After he had checked my heart and blood-pressure he told me that I had nothing to worry about – that my supposedly fatal illness was nothing more serious than a panic attack. This was a very common condition and would explain all the symptoms I had mentioned, he told me. With this reassurance and a strong tranquilliser of some kind which he gave me, I felt much calmer and very relieved. I continued to take tranquillizers over the next three or four weeks, and I didn't have any more trouble.

'Needless to say, the episode left me feeling very shaken and rather foolish. Despite my nursing training, I hadn't heard of panic attacks before, and I didn't realize a psychological problem could be so devastating. I was dismayed when I realized that I hadn't been able to recognize a psychological problem in myself on this occasion. I had been able to do so in the past when I'd had a bout of severe depression, and something approaching agoraphobia on another occasion, when I had taken tranquillizers. It struck me that the doctor didn't have to think too hard to find out the cause of my sudden attack, after all. If he had glanced at my records in his surgery, he would have concluded that I was a bit neurotic anyway.

'That is not to say that I feel "neurotic" all the time. In fact, I've managed to work my way through life quite happily without any serious mental or physical ailments. But I must admit that I may be a bit anxiety-prone. From an early age, I seemed to worry a lot about fainting and making an exhibition of myself in public places, or in case I would become temporarily mad and do something out of the ordinary. As a student nurse, I could be quite absorbed listening to a lecture, and then suddenly I would get the feeling that I was going to pass out and cause a disturbance in class. Even when I was asleep I would sometimes have nightmares in which I found myself in an embarrassing situation. A typical one was that I was back in the sixth form: when I stood up to answer a question, I discovered that I was in my underwear. This sounds very Freudian! The agoraphobic episode occurred about four years before the panic attack and I had almost forgotten it. It didn't mean that I was afraid to go out, but I was afraid to travel on public transport for quite a long time. In retrospect, I think that these various problems were all part and parcel of the same pattern of anxiety, but I can't explain it further than that. I had a very happy and secure childhood, incidentally.

'I think what has helped me most in recent years was that I took up yoga, which has taught me how to relax. This is very important in reducing stress at any time, but it is particularly helpful when you feel you may be working up to a panic attack. There are other ways of learning relaxation and proper breathing patterns, of course. And it is surprising how many people need this kind of help because what happens most of the time when we feel anxious is that we tense up and over-breathe and do all the wrong things.

'If I found myself actually having another panic attack, I would try to relax and follow the advice which Dr Claire Weekes gives in her books, that you shouldn't fight it or try to run away from it or be frightened by it. Instead, you should take slow, deep breaths, and let the unpleasant sensations run through you until they disappear. She calls this "floating" with the panic, and it certainly makes sense to me.'

Kate's account of her own experience covers most of the symptoms listed in the average medical review of the terrifying phenomenon known as panic attack. These include acute apprehension; palpitations and chest pain; breathlessness; dizziness; sweating and trembling; hot and cold flushes; dryness of the mouth; fear of losing control or of dying; a feeling of unreality and a fear of insanity; loss of sensation in limbs; a fear of fainting and general weakness. An episode can last from several minutes to several hours. And, if the condition is not explained and treated, fear of a recurrence can lead to a distressing state of apprehension described as 'chronic anticipatory anxiety'.

The symptoms mentioned are typical of the 'fight or flight' response to stressful situations described earlier. In panic attacks, however, they tend to occur 'out of the blue' at a moment when the sufferer is not aware of being frightened or over-anxious. Because so many of the symptoms seem to coincide in an exceptionally dramatic form, it is not surprising that physical sensations have most impact, especially in a first attack. Kate's doctor had the advantage of seeing her while she was in the grip of an attack, but doctors who see a patient only after an attack has passed can be misled into thinking that some of the symptoms were due to heart trouble: 'As many as one in seven patients who are sent to hospital for cardiological examination are eventually sent down the corridor to the psychiatrist,' Graham Jones wrote in a report on the subject (*General Practitioner*, 4 October 1985).

The background to Kate's sudden attack – a history of

anxiety and phobia (see pages 58-62 and 80-91) – also seems to fit in with the belief held by most European psychiatrists and supported by the World Health Organisation, that the 'panic state' is an acute manifestation of anxiety neurosis which tends to occur suddenly in sensitive individuals with a medical history of anxiety, depression and phobic symptoms of some kind.

On the other hand, American psychiatrists take the view that 'panic disorder' is an entirely different condition with an identity and momentum of its own, and that it requires different treatment from that conventionally given for anxiety. It is clear that Kate's diagnosed panic attack would not be recognized as 'panic disorder' according to the criteria published by the American Psychiatric Association in 1980. Such recognition requires that the patient has had 'At least three panic attacks within a three-week period in circumstances other than during marked physical exertion or in a life-threatening situation' and that 'The disorder is not associated with agoraphobia.' Kate had just one panic attack and she had had agoraphobic symptoms at some time in the past, a not uncommon experience. It seems reasonable to argue, though, that had she not received such prompt attention and reassurance, she might have gone on to suffer further attacks which would satisfy the American criteria for panic disorder.

According to American psychiatrists, about five per cent of the population suffer from true panic disorder at some time in their lives. On this basis, an estimated three million British adults are likely to be affected at any one time, but preliminary findings from a community survey by the Leicester Royal Infirmary, using the American criteria to identify panic disorder among people aged from 16–65 years, have shown a lower prevalence. While nearly 12 per cent of those surveyed had experienced panic attacks, only 3.7 per cent could be said to suffer from panic disorder according to the American criteria, Professor Sydney Brandon reported (*Psychiatry in Practice*, April/May 1986). While the results of such a survey needed to be viewed with caution, he said, they did tend to support the argument that panic disorder is indeed a separate condition.

What the Leicester study also showed was that panic attacks tend to be a much more common occurrence than most people may suspect: 74 people in every 1,000 suffered from panic attacks occasionally, but 23 of these had not had an attack in the previous month. Of those prone to panic, 7 per 1,000 were able to remain panic-free by avoiding situations which they thought might precipitate an attack.

Hyperventilation and its prevention

In some cases recurrence of panic attacks seems to be associated with hyperventilation (over-breathing), and can be controlled by simple training in correct breathing (see pages 73-77). The likelihood that over-breathing can play a crucial role in triggering panic attacks and acute episodes of phobic anxiety has been widely discussed in recent years, both in terms of prevention and self-help treatment.

Breathing is something we do automatically, without ever thinking about it. We start breathing the moment we are born and we stop only when we die. Whatever our understanding of the internal chemistry involved, we know from an early age that the first rule for survival is to keep on breathing.

The rate at which we breathe is another matter of which we are unaware, but which can be speeded up unconsciously when we over-breathe or 'hyperventilate'. Normally, in adult life, we complete the respiratory process involved in breathing in and out at a rate of around 16 or 18 times a minute. When we inhale, we breathe into our lungs air with a 20 per cent oxygen content and a small amount of carbon dioxide; in the lungs, oxygen is picked up by arterial blood and carried to all the tissues of the body. When we exhale, the air we breathe out contains less oxygen, more moisture and a larger proportion of carbon dioxide, a gas formed in the tissues and carried back to the lungs in venous blood.

Over-breathing occurs when, instead of breathing at our normal rate, we take in more air than we need by means of rapid, irregular, sighing breaths, sometimes at a rate of up to 30 in-out breaths a minute, but generally breathing *out* more heavily and *in* only shallowly. We breathe out excessive amounts of carbon dioxide, thus lowering the level of this gas in the blood below that which is normally needed to stimulate breathing. Though hyperventilation and panic attacks sometimes occur after physical exercise, this type of rapid breathing is not to be confused with the ordinary kind of faster breathing involved when we engage in exercise and use up energy at a faster rate than usual.

We all tend to over-breathe to some extent in times of stress. When we do this, we bring about a change in the oxygen-carbon dioxide balance and other chemical changes in the blood which are believed to stimulate our adrenaline out-flow, causing the symptoms like dizziness, palpitations, breathlessness, tingling in the ears and blurred vision so common in panic attacks and acute phobic attacks. Doctors who have studied this phenomenon over many years believe that habitual over-breathing is also responsible for a great many other physical symptoms which doctors find puzzling. These include tension headache, asthma-type illness in patients who do not suffer from asthma, and mysterious conditions like 'total allergy syndrome' and episodes of 'mass hysteria'.

Although over-breathing (hyperventilation syndrome, as it is called) was discussed in a medical report as long ago as 1937, many doctors still discount it as a causal factor in panic attacks. There is no doubt, though, that the condition can cause dizziness and other symptoms common to panic, or that continuous very rapid breathing for more than a few minutes can result in loss of consciousness. The only situation in which deliberate *moderate* over-breathing is encouraged is in a medically supervized 'provocation test': the patient is asked to over-breathe for two or three minutes to see if panic symptoms occur. If they do, it may be assumed that hyperventilation is a feature of that patient's panic attacks, and that training in correct breathing (see pages 73-77) will help to avert further episodes.

The main characteristic of chronic over-breathing is that it is predominantly *thoracic* breathing, which means that respiratory movements are concentrated in the upper part of the chest with only limited movement of the diaphragm, the large dome-shaped muscle separating the chest from

71

the abdominal cavities. Normal breathing tends to combine both thoracic and *abdominal* (diaphragmatic) breathing, so that it is quite natural to alternate deep abdominal breaths with shallow thoracic breaths. It has been noted that men tend to take more deep breaths than women do when at rest and breathing at the normal rate.

While it helps to understand what happens when we breathe normally, it is important for us not to become too preoccupied with our breathing – or any other physical function – when we are feeling perfectly well. The positive and acceptable situation for thinking about the way we breathe is in the context of an exercise programme. The negative and harmful approach is one where we begin to think that the way we normally breathe is wrong somehow, even though we have no symptoms to show for it.

Dr Claude Lum pioneered research into the hyperventilation syndrome and its treatment at Papworth Hospital, Cambridge, in the late 1960s and 1970s. He found that up to 10 per cent of the population may be unconsciously hyperventilating on a fairly regular basis, and consequently experiencing distressing physical symptoms for which their doctors can find no explanation. In studies of over 2,000 patients with the problem, he reported a preponderance of women among younger patients, and of men among those of middle age. Men in this age-group who experience symptoms like palpitations and chest pains due to over-breathing may become unnecessarily fearful of an imminent heart attack. Obviously, a doctor should be consulted without delay in these circumstances, but, as a first-aid measure, it always helps to relax, take the proverbial 'deep breath' and carry out a simple breathing exercise routine (see pages 74-76).

Dr Lum has recorded the successes achieved in the treatment of 1,735 patients with hyperventilation problems that had been confirmed by physiological tests. Over 1,000 of these were given training in relaxation and correct breathing by physiotherapists, with the speed of progress varying according to the severity of symptoms and the patient's age. Many younger patients needed treatment for only a few weeks, while older patients with a more severe problem needed to attend the physiotherapy department for many months before they were free of symptoms. However, twelve months after starting treatment, three-quarters of the group had recovered completely; the remainder took longer to recover or were still experiencing occasional symptoms.

The recommended treatment for severe hyperventilation problems consists both of physiotherapy on an out-patient basis to provide training in breathing control, and of behaviour therapy, especially 'cognitive therapy', which helps the patient to see the symptoms he has experienced in their true light and not in terms of a life-threatening crisis.

Breathing exercises to curb panic and phobic attacks

Physiotherapists are the experts when it comes to assessing and correcting faults involved in the way we breathe, in the way we use our muscles in health and illness, and in the way in which the body's complex network of nerves keeps us functioning efficiently. In recent years, GPs have had the freedom to refer their patients direct to a physiotherapy department where they considered this desirable, so in theory, at least, it should be relatively easy to get an appointment with a physiotherapist. In practice, however, physiotherapists are kept so fully occupied providing treatment for large numbers of patients recovering from serious illnesses or accidents that only those with confirmed and severe hyperventilation problems are likely to be referred to them.

Fortunately, the majority of people who need re-training to overcome a habit of over-breathing associated with milder and occasional episodes of anxiety and panic can be guided towards self-help. For instance, in a panic attack, our natural impulse usually is to try to fight it and retain control over the situation at all costs, whereas the easiest way to regain composure is to relax and let the frightening feelings burn themselves out. For most people with a moderate problem, the best approach is likely to be a programme of breathing re-training exercises, combined with membership of a self-help group in which the principles of correct breathing and behaviour therapy are understood.

The essential aim of breathing re-training exercises is to change over from a pattern of mainly thoracic (upper chest) breathing with rapid, shallow, sighing and irregular breaths, to a pattern of predominantly diaphragmatic (with abdominal movement) breathing, which is slower, deeper and regular. If an episode of over-breathing is anticipated, starting with dizziness and other symptoms of a panic attack, the sufferer can manage to cope with it by doing the exercises. The following routine is based on Dr Claude Lum's programme:

> Sit in a comfortable chair and relax so that your muscles go limp and your limbs feel heavy. Imagine that you are resting on a sunny beach. Take a deep breath, filling your lungs with air so that you can feel movement below the belt-line in your abdominal muscles. Continue to breathe in and out deeply and regularly at a rate of about 12 intakes of breath a minute, while counting by the second hand of a watch or clock. Continue with the exercise until you feel completely calm. (If you start the exercises feeling very panicky with noticeably rapid and irregular breathing, you may need to 'over-correct' your breathing by taking only 8 breaths a minute for a few minutes to restore the level of carbon dioxide in your respiration.)

Another simple self-help first-aid exercise to counteract panic feelings (by restoring the carbon-dioxide/oxygen balance which is disrupted by over-breathing) is taught by specialists at St Bartholomew's Hospital, London, who have studied the problem of hyperventilation in relation to panic attacks. This is particularly useful if you feel symptoms coming on when you are in a public place:

> If possible, find a seat. If there is none available in the vicinity, lean your back against a wall and try to relax. Now bring your hands close together and cup

them around your mouth and nose, so that you are breathing in expired air which contains much more carbon dioxide than ordinary air. Breathe in and out deeply and evenly until the panic feelings subside. You can also use a paper bag instead of cupped hands. However, using your hands has the advantage that it is unlikely to attract attention.

One of the most successful programmes for bringing faulty breathing under control and cutting short the frightening symptoms of a panic or phobic attack has been developed by Dr Claire Weekes. For anyone who has ever experienced a panic attack or phobic attack, her slogan, 'Float and not fight', makes good sense. The more we resist and consciously try to fight the symptoms, the more we are re-triggering the chemical mechanisms which cause the panic to continue. 'If, instead, you relax and let the frightening feelings run through you, they will disappear all the more quickly,' she promises. Her technique is based on four principles: facing, accepting, floating, letting time pass. The following is a condensed version of these principles:

Facing the fear and not running away from it: Sit as comfortably as you can by letting your arms and legs sag into the chair as if charged with lead. Take slow, deep breaths through your partly opened mouth. Now examine in your mind each of the upsetting sensations. Do not shrink from them. Describe each symptom aloud to yourself and analyse it. For example, "My hands sweat and tremble." Relax.'

Accepting: 'True acceptance is the keystone to recovery. For example, be prepared to let your stomach churn while you go on reading a newspaper. Then, freed from the stimulus of tension and anxiety, the adrenaline-releasing nerves will calm down, and the churning will automatically lessen and will finally cease.'

Floating instead of fighting involves 'masterly

inactivity' and letting go: 'It means to give up the struggle, to stop holding tensely on to yourself, trying to control your fear. Don't strive for relaxation. Wait for it. Recognize that there is no battle to fight except one of your own making. If you feel paralysed by fear, don't force yourself to fight your way into shops and public transport. Instead, imagine that you are completely relaxed and floating on a cloud, and just float in. Floating relaxes tension and makes it easy to take action.'

Letting time pass means not being impatient if your progress seems slower than you had hoped. Keep yourself occupied but not obsessively so. It means taking sedative medication if you need it: 'You need not fear addiction from supervized sedation . . . so many patients try to do without it too soon.' It takes time also to get rid of apprehension: 'It is comforting to know that the action of adrenaline is always restricted to the same organs, and so must always follow the same pattern. There are no surprises in store for you.'

A great many people are fortunate enough to go through life without ever learning what it means to have a panic attack. Many others are lucky enough to have only one solitary attack, even if the fear it generates lingers on for a long time. But for many others less fortunate, a first frightening attack may be only the beginning of a nightmare, in which 'fear of fear' (phobophobia, as the experts call it) is a constant reminder that there may well be a next time. Yet this fear can also be conquered. Understanding what causes an attack, and the chemical mechanisms which can give rise to so many distressing symptoms, is the best way of ensuring that there won't be a next time.

Drawing on the wisdom gained through years of professional experience, Dr Weekes counsels against impatience. We must not lose hope if the threat of fear is not conquered completely 'overnight'. We also need to 'let time pass' for the healing process to take root and bring recovery after any traumatic experience, and emotional crises are no exception. It is, as she reminds us, a comforting thought that for those who have endured one panic attack, a recurrence holds no further surprises. To have an attack is to learn the hard way that this is not a prelude to loss of control or madness or sudden death. It is equally reassuring to know that an attack can be prevented by the time-honoured expedient of relaxing and taking a deep breath.

Drug treatments for anxiety and panic
For many years, tranquillizers in the benzodiazepine group have been considered the most effective treatment for general anxiety and mild panic attacks. Benzodiazepine compounds form the main group of *minor* tranquillizers, and are entirely different from the *major* tranquillizers (see pages 141-143) which are given for psychotic illnesses such as schizophrenia. Benzodiazepines act in four ways: as an anti-anxiety drug; as a sedative; as a muscle relaxant; and as an anti-convulsant. Because of the latter effect, some of them are also used to treat epilepsy.

These tranquillizers come under four different headings: long-acting and medium-acting tranquillizers; long-acting and medium-acting hypnotics (sleeping pills). Many of them can cause drowsiness, especially in the early stages. They can also cause confusion in elderly people, which may be mistaken for symptoms of dementia. All of these drugs can affect judgement and manual dexterity, and a warning to patients to this effect is necessary if they are car-drivers or work with potentially dangerous machinery.

In the following lists of minor tranquillizers and sleeping pills in frequent use, drugs are identified by their British trade names.

Long-acting tranquillizers (diazepam, clorazepate, etc.): Alupram, Anxon, Atensive, Centrax, Diazemuls, Evacalm, Frisium, Lexotan, Librium, Nobrium, Stesolid, Solis, Tensium, Tranxene, Tropium, Valium, Valrelease.

Medium-acting tranquillizers (oxazepam, lorazepam, etc.): Almazine, Ativan, Oxanid, Serenid-D, Xanax.

Long-acting sleeping pills (hitrazepam, flurazepam, etc.): Dalmane, Mogadon, Nitrados, Noctesed, Remnos, Rohypnol, Somnite, Surem, Unisomnia.

Medium-acting sleeping pills (temazepam, lormetazepam, etc.): Euhypnos, Loramet, Normison, Noctamid.

Barbiturates
These 'controlled drugs' are no longer prescribed for anxiety but are limited to the treatment of patients with special problems, such as intractable insomnia. They include Amytal, Phanodorm, Nembutal, Seconal, Soneryl.

When taken according to instructions, benzodiazepines usually have few adverse side-effects apart from drowsiness and perhaps some initial unsteadiness due to the muscle-relaxant effects of the drug. It should be remembered that these drugs interact with alcohol and other drugs, such as anti-depressants which have a depressing effect on the central nervous system. Doctors are advised, however, to exercise caution in prescribing benzodiazepines for certain groups of people: the elderly; women during pregnancy, labour and lactation; sufferers from certain respiratory conditions; and patients with chronic kidney or liver disease.

Long-term use should be avoided, and the drug should be withdrawn gradually by reducing the daily dose over several weeks, to avoid troublesome withdrawal symptoms. Only a relatively small proportion of tranquillizer users are believed to be at risk of severe withdrawal symptoms (which can include anxiety, depression and panic symptoms) and these tend to be people on large doses for a long period who stop the drug too abruptly.

Very rarely, benzodiazepines can *cause* an increase in symptoms such as anxiety and depression in the early stages of treatment. Where this happens, the patient should report back promptly to the doctor, and is likely to find that a different member of the drug group will have a beneficial effect.

Because of recent evidence that benzodiazepines have been over-prescribed for excessive lengths of time, and the realization that prolonged use can lead to dependence, their benefits are sometimes forgotten. In *Psychiatry in Practice* (April/May 1986), Surrey GP Dr Richard France commented: 'It is ironic that more effort is going into developing techniques for the withdrawal of tranquillizers than into finding new ways of treating the anxiety for which they were previously prescribed.'

However, a leading British authority, Professor Malcolm Lader of London University, leaves his medical readers in no doubt that benzodiazepines remain the 'treatments of choice for anxiety' (*GP*, 6 September 1985).

Professor Lader's scheme for the management of anxiety has as its starting point, support, reassurance and practical advice for the patient, with the involvement of relatives and friends. In a case of *mild to moderate anxiety*, reassurance without medication is recommended as the initial approach to treatment. If symptoms persist, then a benzodiazepine is advocated, but in the minimum dosage needed for the desired effect; and if the response to this is satisfactory, the drug should be prescribed for a few weeks only. On the other hand, if distressing nervous and physical symptoms remain troublesome, a beta-blocker drug may be given as an extra or substitute measure. Beta-blockers such as propranolol achieve their calming effect by blocking nervous stimulation, so that blood-pressure is lowered and the heart's response to stress is reduced. Therefore, doctors have to be extra careful in prescribing these drugs.

In *severe anxiety*, treatment starts off with a benzodiazepine combined with behavioural or psychoanalytic psychotherapy. Frequent reviews are recommended, and the drug is withdrawn gradually if there are signs of tolerance or dependence. If symptoms remain severely disabling without such treatment, a benzodiazepine is continued for as long as the benefits outweigh the risk of drug dependence. In all cases where symptoms fail to respond to the drug, the doctor is advised to check that the patient is taking medication correctly and regularly as prescribed.

In Britain and the United States, the standard treatment for *panic disorder* usually consists of anti-depressants in the tricyclic and MAOI groups (see pages 142-143), combined with behaviour therapy or participation in an effective self-help programme. Many British doctors also favour these drugs for patients having an isolated panic attack, and those with a history of depression.

These regimens obviously are a far cry from the indiscriminate and prolonged use of tranquillizers which has been the subject of so many serious complaints. One of our main safeguards against developing dependence on tranquillizers or any other potentially addictive drugs is that we take some of the responsibility into our own hands. We don't have to go on asking for repeat prescriptions by the simple process of leaving a note in the surgery. If the symptoms are not substantially improved after one repeat prescription, then it is time to see the doctor again. It is also important to remember that these drugs should not be stopped suddenly, because of the risk of withdrawal symptoms; they should be reduced gradually over several weeks under medical supervision.

PHOBIC ANXIETY

A phobia is an irrational or exaggerated fear which has a disturbing effect on a person's life out of proportion to its cause. It has been estimated that over half a million British people suffer from a severe form of the disorder, experiencing recurrent phobic attacks: these are essentially panic attacks with the additional component of a specific fear of some kind. A much larger number of people suffer from a milder form of phobia in which the object or situation feared can more easily be avoided, and in which panic attacks are rare.

Phobic anxiety is not a condition which can be considered on its own as totally distinct from other forms of neurotic illness: both reactive and endogenous depression may activate phobic or obsessional behaviour, according to consultant psychiatrist Dr Colin Brewer (*GP*, 28 February 1986). Professor Isaac Marks of the Institute of Psychiatry, London, suggests that all anxiety symptoms can be summarized in terms of six overlapping syndromes:

- generalized anxiety
- anxiety and panic attacks

- panic
- phobia – simple or social with or without panic attacks
- agoraphobia without panic
- agoraphobia with panic.

Various methods of classification have been developed to distinguish between different types of phobia. One approach divides phobias initially into three broad categories according to the nature of the fear: fear of a specific animal or object; fear of a particular place or situation; fear of an abstract kind, such as dread of an illness or fear of death.

Yet another system for understanding phobias involves considering them as forming discernible groups.

Animal phobias (including birds, insects and snakes) often start in childhood, usually before the age of six and the majority of sufferers are women.

Social phobias (starting in adolescence or early adult life and affecting equal numbers of men and women) include fear of blushing, speaking, eating or drinking when others are present.

Single-symptom phobias (common to both men and women) can begin at any time of life and include fear of darkness, heights, thunderstorms.

Illness phobias (fear of cancer, heart disease, sexually transmitted diseases and death) are common to both men and women and usually start in middle age.

Agoraphobia (the most common severe phobias, involving fear of public places) affects at least twice as many women as men; symptoms usually develop between the ages of 15 and 35, and in later years often coincide with difficulties in a marital relationship.

Claustrophobia (an oppressive fear of being unable to escape from a confined space such as a lift or an underground train) affects both men and women.

Most of us have some 'pet aversion' about which we are mildly phobic without the feeling ever reaching the dimensions of an emotional problem. Research has shown that some people can develop phobias involving concepts as apparently innocuous as rain (ombrophobia), string (linonophobia) or wind (anemophobia). But it is not difficult to imagine how, in certain circumstances, one might develop a phobia focused on potentially frightening situations like sleep, dreams, being buried alive, submerged in water or lost in darkness, to mention just a few possible triggering factors on the experts' list.

Marion's dread of water dates back to early childhood in the war years, when she had a recurrent dream of water rising rapidly around her bed. Her mother remembers how she would wake up screaming, still convinced that she could see water rising. Terrifying dreams in her teens led to Angela's dread of falling asleep and losing control, which took many years to overcome completely: 'It started after a sudden death in the family and eased off only when I was in my mid-twenties,' she recalls. 'The dreams were so horrifying that they seemed more real than reality while they lasted. I got various pills to help get over the bump of anxiety about dropping off to sleep, but nothing helped for long. So for years I just read one detective story after another, waiting for sheer exhaustion to knock me out.'

Obviously, some simple phobias are easy to live with by avoiding the source of fear. Sylvia's dread of 'creepy-crawlies' began one summer day in early childhood when she was playing beside a tilled garden. An older sister said, 'Shut your eyes and open your hands and see what God will send you.' Sylvia went into an 'hysterical fit', she recalls, when she found out that the pretended gift was a handful of wriggling earthworms and snails. Now in her twenties and living in the city, she manages to avoid seeing these harmless creatures most of the time, but 'I couldn't possibly take up a hobby like gardening – the very suspicion of something crawling anywhere near me is enough to send me into a shivering fit and I want to be sick,' she says.

Some phobias cannot be easily avoided, such as the fear of illness, which has its roots in the sufferer's own thoughts. In other cases, such as social phobias and agoraphobia, avoiding the source of fear can in fact create problems which are far more incapacitating than the fear itself. 'Avoidance' is an important medical term summing up the lengths to which many sufferers feel compelled to go to escape from a feared situation, while also pointing the way to treatment where the fear can be faced and gradually conquered.

One fear which we all find it easy to identify and sympathize with is claustrophobia, as Dr Joyce Emerson confirmed in her 1969 Family Doctor booklet, *Phobias*: 'Most people seem to be able to imagine how one can feel afraid of being shut in, even if they don't themselves suffer from this fear . . . People suffering from claustrophobia often insist on sitting at the end of a row or near an exit in the cinema or theatre, or on sleeping with their bedroom door open. In this way they feel that they could get out easily if necessary.' Many people who are not recognizably claustrophobic often behave in this way, of course; no doubt most of these have anxieties which they manage to keep in perspective otherwise. Jean's friends know that she has 'a thing' about sitting on end seats even in underground trains, and can get 'quite paranoid' if someone presses her to take a seat in the centre of the train. Yet, paradoxically, she has to sleep with her bedroom door locked because she is terrified of being awakened by an intruder. Conversely, her sister, Carol, can sleep only if the door is wide open 'to let in fresh air'. Both lead perfectly normal lives, but their mother was subject to panic attacks for some years. Anxiety in different forms does tend to run in families, something many authorities see as the result of 'learned behaviour'. Recent research suggests that the explanation may instead be found in some delicate anomaly in body biochemistry affecting the metabolism of some food substances.

The commonest and, in severe cases, the most disabling form of phobia is agoraphobia, a Greek word which literally means 'fear of the market place'. About 60 per cent of all phobics with a severe problem are agoraphobics, and over two-thirds of them are women. Very often the sufferer tries to cope by remaining indoors and becoming housebound, unless the right kind of help is at hand. 'An agoraphobic is typically a child of parents who are themselves, one or both of them, phobic to some degree,' say Dr Fredric Neuman, associate director of the famous White Plains Hospital Phobia Clinic in New York. While conceding the possibility that a genetic vulnerability to the illness may be inherited in some cases, he believes that a major part is played by 'contagion of ideas' in families where fear and anxiety is prevalent. What is certain, he adds, is that somehow in the process of growing up, the phobic develops certain misconceptions about himself and about the world which form the basis of the illness. The sufferer regards the world as fundamentally a dangerous place, and physical health as a precarious matter, ideas likely to have been acquired in childhood.

Dr Neuman acquired an active interest in phobias and agoraphobia in particular when, as a student, he became phobic himself: 'One day without any evident reason I became panicky. I had the feeling I was going to go crazy or scream or in some way lose control of myself. It was a dramatic and inexplicable feeling. It was obvious, I thought, that something terrible was the matter with me. After leafing through the pages of my college psychology textbook, I tentatively decided I was suffering from an anxiety reaction, a neurotic depression probably, a panic attack also, and a variety of other illnesses – possibly including schizophrenia. In the opinion of my room-mate, I was also a hypochondriac.' Young Fredric Neuman would have consulted a psychiatrist at the outset had he not feared that a record of emotional illness might prejudice his chances of admission to medical school. Although a doctor assured him that there was no need to worry unless he also had a 'character disorder', he was not convinced: 'I naturally assumed that I had a character disorder, whatever that was, along with everything else. So I lived with the condition for the next few years – with considerable difficulty as everyone does – and along the way stumbled over the principles of treatment that allowed me finally to get well.'

Most serious phobias are variants of agorophobia, Dr Neuman argues. And phobias merge into each other, so that someone who is afraid to drive over bridges is also likely to be afraid of travelling on buses and planes, shopping in supermarkets, or attending elaborate social events. On the other hand, simple phobias like fear of snakes or fear of flying can occur in isolation, without interfering with the sufferer's life so long as the source of fear is avoided. We all know perfectly well-adjusted people who confess to being terrified of spiders, after all.

There are cases, however, where the diagnosis and treatment of a severe phobia can present difficulties because the phobia is only one symptom of an emotional illness, says Professor Marks, who is a leading researcher and writer on this subject.

Phobias occurring on their own are, in severe cases, classified as phobic disorders. But where a phobia is a feature of an existing condition, such as depressive illness, generalized anxiety, obsession or compulsive disorder (see pages 91-96) , priority is given to treating the underlying problem, thus automatically relieving the phobic symptoms. When phobia is a complication of depression, for instance, it tends to fluctuate in severity in keeping with the sufferer's mood changes, and usually improves when an effective anti-depressant is given.

While Dr Neuman's American experience has led him to believe that 'contagion' of fearful ideas and parental anxiety often predispose to agoraphobia later in the child's life, Professor Marks stresses that most sufferers come from stable families. But perhaps these claims are less of a contradiction than might appear at first glance since even the most stable people can be prone to anxiety. As in the case of other emotional disorders, agoraphobia often develops after some major event or change in the sufferer's life, such as a bereavement, leaving home, miscarriage or childbirth. It has been noted that many women develop agoraphobia after marriage, in response to some (usually unexpressed) dissatisfaction with the marital relationship. It is not unusual, however, for sufferers to attribute the start of their trouble to some trivial event which they would not normally find disturbing, possibly indicating that they were already feeling emotionally fragile before some 'last straw' triggered a phobic attack.

A cure for phobias

The good news about phobias is that they are curable. In rare cases, recovery occurs very rapidly; in the majority of cases it occurs over a period of months; and in some severe cases it may take a year or longer. The key to recovery is a self-help programme based on a clear understanding of the problem and undertaken with the guidance of a doctor, therapist or recognized self-help group. But before any of this can happen, the sufferer must be prepared to admit that she needs help and to speak openly about her fears and other symptoms, so as to avoid delay in starting the correct treatment.

If you have recently developed symptoms which you think may be due to a severe form of anxiety or phobia, then the first person to see is your own doctor. Equally, you should encourage sufferers known to you to do the same. This is essential both to make sure that you are not suffering from some physical ailment which needs treatment, and because your GP is the only person who can refer you for specialist treatment under the National Health Service, if this is necessary. Fortunately, most GPs understand a great deal more about psychological problems than is sometimes thought, and nowadays it often happens that a successful behaviour therapy programme can be arranged by the patient's own doctor, with the assistance of a community psychiatric nurse or specialist social worker (see page 170).

Communication between you and the doctor is crucially important. You must be prepared to come to grips with the real purpose of your visit, and to realize that it is neither silly nor shameful, nor at all exceptional, to have to confess to phobic symptoms. Such feelings, according to doctors, often create a barrier to communication, and result in inappropriate treatment and further loss of confidence for the patient.

Whether or not drugs are prescribed depends on your present symptoms and recent medical history. If you were previously troubled by anxiety or depression or sleep disturbance, the doctor may decide that you can be helped by a prescription for a minor tranquillizer or anti-depressant. While there is some controversy about the usefulness of drugs in treating phobias, their value in treating an underlying depression associated with a phobia is recognized, especially where behaviour therapy is also provided.

Behaviour therapy is the form of psychotherapy found to be most successful in the shortest period of time in bringing relief to phobia sufferers. What does it involve, and how does it differ from analytic psychotherapy, which is widely used in many forms of mental disorder?

Behaviour therapy is based on the assumption that harmful attitudes and behaviours such as those seen in phobias have been learned, and therefore can be un-learned and altered, so that the sufferer develops a positive outlook. The full understanding and cooperation of the patient are essential, since the success of therapy depends on her willingness to face up to her own fears, under professional guidance.

The main focus of attention in behaviour therapy is the patient's current problem in the 'here and now', rather than the question as to why she developed a phobia in the first place. However, in dealing with very difficult problems, behaviour therapists usually include elements of the more exploratory analytic psychotherapy to help patients gain a deeper insight into the background to their illness. Behaviour therapy also has the advantage that the techniques used to treat phobias are relatively easy to teach to GPs, nurses and social workers and, of course, to patients and their relatives and leaders of self-help groups.

Analytic psychotherapy is a development of psychoanalysis, which derives its authority from Sigmund Freud's theory that the explanation for disturbed behaviour and many mental disorders is to be found in events which occurred in early childhood and especially in those involving the mother-child relationship. Through a psychoanalytic approach, the patient is helped to explore past experiences stored in the unconscious mind, and thus to understand – and cope with – the emotional damage which may have resulted from some apparently forgotten traumatic event.

The disadvantages of this approach are that it is slow, time-consuming and expensive, and less successful in achieving rapid improvement in phobic patients: it calls for the participation of highly skilled therapists who have completed a recognized course of training and involve regular weekly sessions for a year or longer. Consequently, analytic psychotherapy tends to be less readily available under the National Health Service than behaviour therapy.

Exposure therapy is the form of behaviour therapy found to be most successful in treating phobias. It is basically a behaviour modification technique which involves gradually 'exposing' the patient to an object or situation which she has been avoiding because of the distress it causes. In this way she comes to learn that she can remain in a frightening situation without any danger or embarrassment to herself, and in time she loses her fear of it. In treating spider phobia, for instance, the patient is helped to relax and in successive sessions is asked to imagine a spider in a variety of different situations, then to progress to looking at pictures of spiders, and finally to look at and perhaps even touch a real spider.

Again, to be successful, exposure therapy requires the patient to be completely cooperative in carrying out a carefully structured programme of exposure exercises, and in keeping a diary record of 'homework'. An example of an agoraphobic diary from Professor Isaac Marks' clinic includes the following entries: 'Wednesday: Walked to local supermarket and surrounding shops, bought food and presents for family, visited café. Comments: Felt worse when shops were crowded, practised deep-breathing exercises. *Friday*: Rode a bus to town and back three times till I felt better about it. Comments: Worst when bus was crowded – did deep-breathing exercises.' In this case the patient's husband acted as co-therapist and signed the record to show that the tasks had been completed (*MIMS Magazine*, 15 February 1985).

'The great majority of compliant sufferers can lose most of their fears within a few weeks, provided that they are willing to work hard in an exposure programme, Professor Marks explains. 'Exposure treatment involves the phobic deliberately entering the fear-evoking situation, staying there until the anxiety starts to subside, and repeating the exercise many times until what formerly evoked terror has now become merely boring. In most patients it takes at least half an hour before the fear begins to decrease and several hours before it diminishes to the point where the patient has lost a substantial part of the handicap. A few patients get better so quickly that it takes them some time to realize that they are no longer phobic. Improvement is faster if the exposure sessions last for two hours rather than for shorter periods of time… After successful exposure treatment, improvement tends to continue up to the four- to seven-year follow-ups that have been carried out in several countries.'

Dr Fredric Neuman has devised an eight-stage programme for recovery from a severe phobia which forms the basis of the eight-week session of exposure therapy at his clinic.

The first stage helps the *diagnosed* patient to recognize that he has a phobia and to understand how it affects his life. He is asked to make detailed notes of situations which induce panic for him and those which are least stressful, and then to construct a 'hierarchy of fear', in which the least frightening situations are listed at the bottom and the most frightening appear at the top. This information makes it possible to plan exposure, so that more difficult tasks are approached by easy stages while fear is being overcome gradually.

In stage two, the patient enters into a commitment of 'being willing to try'. He learns how exposure therapy works and about the successes it has achieved. The third stage concentrates on 'being open and working with others', stressing the importance of joining a self-help group and finding someone in the family or social circle to act in the role of 'helper' or 'co-therapist' under the guidance of a professional therapist.

Stage four is headed 'Practising – just a few feet farther, just a little while longer'. Here Dr Neuman emphasizes the role of planning in the programme and of 'proper pacing', so that the patient understands the amount of time to be spent on exposure therapy 'homework' tasks every day, and the rate at which improvement is expected to proceed. Patients begin with less difficult tasks at the bottom of their hierarchy of fears, but go a little further and stay a little longer each day. There are also encouraging reminders that some phobics who worry for days about tackling a particular task find that their anxiety evaporates when the time for action arrives, and, importantly, that inability to complete a given task should not be regarded as a failure. 'There is no shame in starting and stopping. Someone who feels that every plan he makes must be executed exactly will be afraid of making ambitious plans and soon will not want to practise at all.'

In stage five the programme comes to grips with the patient's need to be able to cope with episodes of increasing anxiety and panic attacks: 'There is one key to management, and it is perhaps the fundamental principle of treatment. Do not wait passively. Do something. Assert control of yourself by acting upon your environment. Take hold of your thoughts and feelings. Talk to the person in front of you about anything. Add up in your mind the prices of purchases you wish to make. Write a letter. Occupy yourself with counting backwards from one hundred, chew a piece of gum, play with your car keys. And keep a written record of the incident.'

By stage six the tasks will have become more difficult and may have to be broken down into smaller 'do-able' pieces before they can be completed for the first time. For example, getting past 'stuck points' for someone frightened of using an escalator can be achieved by carrying out eight simple steps, starting with observing other users and gaining confidence from their calmness, then imagining oneself on the escalator, then proceeding with the support of a helper to the point where it is possible to move up and down on the escalator without undue concern. By stages seven and eight, the patient is likely to be feeling much better and improving at a faster pace, and will finally be in a position to plan ahead for a panic-free future.

The value of behaviour therapy in treating phobic and obsessional disorders is stressed by Dr Richard Stern, consultant psychiatrist, St Anthony's Hospital, Surrey. In response to critics who said, 'These treatments are dangerous, patients will go psychotic' or 'These treatments are superficial. You have to treat the underlying cause or else other symptoms emerge,' he cites numerous studies which prove these criticisms to be unfounded. 'Patients given behaviour therapy under skilled guidance do not go psychotic, do not develop other symptoms, nor do they relapse.' Nor should his views be interpreted as an attack on Freudian thought or psychoanalysis: 'Freud himself was most "unfreudian" in his methods, often exhorting his patients to get up from the couch and venture out into the phobic situation!' As Dr Stern remarks, behaviour therapy has brought about a revolution not only in the treatment of patients but also in the behaviour of therapists: 'Prior to 1950 it was very unusual for a psychiatrist to leave his chair and take an agoraphobic patient for a walk.'

OBSESSIONS AND COMPULSIONS
Most of us have indulged in mildly obsessive behaviour at some time without being any the worse for it. Superstitious observances learned in childhood most often account for the way in which we perform harmless rituals as a defence against misfortune. Preoccupation with numbers is almost universal in moments of anxiety, for instance: 'If I don't carry out this action three times, something awful will happen.' Or, conversely, 'If I do this three times, I can prevent some terrible catastrophe.' Who hasn't heard and sometimes believed the old saying that misfortunes come in threes, for example, and that you can break the spell: if you accidentally break two treasured pieces of bric-a-brac, you should get in first and smash something of little value. And who has not at some time felt compelled to step on or between the joins in paving-stones? So it could be said that when obsessive-compulsive behaviour takes on the dimensions of a neurotic illness, it is only a case of feelings

91

which are common to all of us getting out of control for some reason.

Severe phobias and obsessive-compulsive disorders have many similarities. Both can produce dramatic changes in behaviour which have a disruptive effect on the sufferer's lifestyle. Avoidance of frightening objects or situations is a shared characteristic but the most obvious difference is the obsessive patient's compulsion to counteract the effects of fear by repeatedly carrying out certain rituals, such as hand-washing to avoid contamination. Both conditions respond favourably to behaviour therapy.

A telling demonstration of the relationship between phobias and obsessive-compulsive disorders was given over 20 years ago by F. Kraupl Taylor: 'An anxiety neurotic patient with a phobia of dirt takes good care to keep away from anything dirty, and if he has been in touch with a dirty object is driven by his panic to cleanse himself immediately and thoroughly. An obsessive-compulsive person with a similar phobia has to keep away even from objects that look scrupulously clean because the mere thought that they are dirty may magically make them dirty and also contaminate him even if he cannot remember having touched them.'

Obsessional fears can take many forms, Professor Anthony Clare says: 'The obsessional may, for example, be terrified by the fear that he will shout obscenities in church, take his clothes off in public, injure himself or others, make indecent suggestions to strangers, or throw himself off high buildings or in front of moving vehicles.' One of the commonest manifestations of the disorder is, however, fear of some form of contamination, which drives the sufferer to resort to interminable hand-washing. Various theories have been suggested to explain the psychological basis for this particular type of compulsion. One is that it dates back to early toilet training and a fear of dirt fostered by parental reminders to 'Go and wash your hands.'

Another theory has it that the compulsive hand-washer is responding to an unconscious urge to wash away a sense of guilt for real or imagined sins, in the tradition of Pontius Pilate or Shakespeare's Lady Macbeth, or that scrubbing the hands has a certain natural symbolism when we feel the need to rid ourselves of unpleasant memories or impressions. Since many of those affected by this particular problem are conscientious and highly sensitive adolescents who take their responsibilities very seriously, this is not such a far-fetched idea as it may seem.

Philip, an O-level student, was a teenager in this mould who took his religious education very much to heart, and was therefore dismayed to find his mind often harbouring 'impure thoughts' which he could not control. He felt there was no one in whom he could confide, and no one observed any outward symptoms of his conflict until his fear of dirt reached the stage where his preoccupation with bathing and hand-washing was apparent to everyone in his family. For Philip, this was the beginning of regular sessions with a psychiatrist over several years. Although he may already have been vulnerable, Philip believes that the catalyst which preceded his plunge into obsessional neurosis was a visit to the cinema where he saw an old film version of Oscar Wilde's story, *The Portrait of Dorian Gray*. This depicts the evil career of a dissolute young man who sells his soul in exchange for the gift of eternal youth and good looks. A condition of the bargain is that he keep hidden in his home a self-portrait which will show as the years pass all the ravages of ageing and depravity which he personally is spared. It is not difficult to imagine how a highly sensitive youth might identify with the subject, and become deeply disturbed when the portrait finally emerges to reveal the hideous marks of an inordinately lengthy and sinful life.

Not all obsessional problems are so easily recognized, however, and, fortunately, not all are so difficult to treat. When sixteen-year-old Dorothy saw her doctor because of a troublesome rash on her hands and forearms, she did not think of mentioning the fact that she had been using an antiseptic solution to scrub these areas many times a day for several months. She was convinced that the problem was due to infection and, when several remedies were tried and failed, she was referred to a hospital dermatologist. It was only after detailed questioning that her frequent hand-washing practices came to light, and she was referred back to her own GP for reassessment. It transpired that the problem had set in following a frightening incident in a public park when she was accosted by a man from whom she managed to escape after a struggle. The encounter left her feeling shocked and unclean and irrationally guilty for having in some unknown way attracted the man's attention. Dorothy was able to make a full recovery after she had been treated by a clinical psychologist for several months.

'Washing serves to reduce anxiety, and so tends to reinforce continued washing,' according to Dr Stern. He described the case of a woman patient whose obsessive fear was that she would pass on a cancer 'germ' to her family by touching them (*MIMS Magazine*, 1 October 1980). 'In her own mind she connected spreading cancer with the fact that she had been told warts could be spread by touching someone who had a wart. Therefore she washed her hands 125 times a day, used three bars of soap a day, took three hours to shower, and washed her hair repeatedly for fear of contamination by a cancer-causing "germ". She realized that cancer could not be "caught" in this way but gave way to washing rituals because, in her own words, "I feel a great sense of relief when I've carried out a thorough wash to my own satisfaction." An irrational fear of spreading cancer has led to her avoiding physical contact with other people and to excessive washing . . . Exacerbating factors include contact with her parents, because her greatest fear is of giving cancer to them. For this reason, she refuses to prepare or cook meals for her parents.'

Because of the severity of her problem, Dr Stern's patient was admitted to hospital for behaviour therapy, which began by limiting her use of soap to one bar a day. By supervizing her during washing and preventing her from washing under a running tap, the staff were able to bring about a gradual decrease in the number of washes she had each day and the time spent on them. One technique used by the therapist with the aim of weaning the patient away from her obsession was to 'contaminate' her by persuading her to touch objects used by a large number of people, such as door knobs. After 47 treatment sessions, the patient was using only one bar of soap every two weeks, and was able to return to work. At a follow-up interview a year later, she was found to be keeping well.

While for some people compulsive actions are the main manifestation of an obsessive disorder, for others the overwhelming problem takes the form of persistent irrational and disturbing thoughts. Obsessive ruminations, as these thoughts are called, often are an exaggerated version of everyday 'worrying'. One of Dr Stern's patients, a 27-year-old man, had been worrying in a 'ruminative' way for about ten years about such actions as turning off taps or the car ignition. He hardly ever went back to check on his actions but his anxiety increased gradually over the years until by the time he sought treatment he was finding it impossible to concentrate on his work.

This patient's successful treatment included 15 therapy sessions (three 45-minute sessions a week), each starting with relaxation. The man was asked to make a list of his obsessional fears and, starting with the least severe of these, he was asked to imagine himself carrying out one of the actions which worried him, such as turning off a tap. When he had done this in imagination, he was asked to worry about it for up to 15 seconds and raise his hand when he had visualized his obsessional fear. At this point the therapist tapped sharply on the desk and the patient was told to shout 'stop' simultaneously. At the word 'stop', the obsessional thought should disappear, and it always did so. In time, the patient found that he could use this technique effectively in his everyday life, and that he could cope with his work again.

'Thought-stopping' and 'satiation therapy' are two of the newer techniques used in behaviour therapy for obsessive thoughts. Dr Stern stresses the importance in the early stages of treatment of the patient's saying 'stop' out loud to coincide with a sharp noise. Later on he can give himself the instruction more quietly until he can control obsessive thoughts by saying the word inaudibly. Obviously, this is a method we could all learn to use against the destructive (though non-obsessional) depressing thoughts which have a nasty habit of creeping up on us from time to time.

95

A dictionary definition of the word 'satiation' is 'satisfaction' or 'weariness caused through over-fulfilment'. The latter definition applies more accurately to satiation therapy, a technique often found to be helpful where thought-stopping is ineffective. As Dr Stern explains, it approaches the problem from the opposite extreme and could be compared with the use of exposure therapy. 'Obsessional thoughts [ruminations] must be distinguished from obsessional actions [compulsions or rituals], as each requires a separate treatment approach. Here the aim is to teach the patient to face his abhorrent rumination and think about it for prolonged periods until the rumination abates.'

As Dr Stern stresses, behaviour therapy involves the use of potent techniques and for this reason, and to obtain the most favourable results, *treatment should only be provided by therapists with a recognized qualification*. This is just as true for psychoanalytic psychotherapy, hypnotherapy and the many other forms of therapy which are now on offer. In the absence of a clear-cut professional registration system, it is always wise to seek authoritative advice before making private arrangements to consult a therapist who is unknown to you.

HYSTERIA

The popular view of hysteria tends to centre on the image of the 'hysterical woman', an overgrown spoilt child of an excitable, impulsive, attention-seeking disposition who is given to histrionic outbursts when things don't go her way. Indeed, these are the sort of characteristics which doctors include in a description of the 'hysterical personality'. Initially doctors thought that only women suffered from the malady, that its symptoms were due to the loosening of the womb from its pelvic attachments: the term 'hysteria' means 'pertaining to the womb'.

The study of hysteria is now divided into three broad categories:
conversion hysteria, affecting both men and women, in which emotional stress is 'converted' into a physical disability such as blindness or paralysis.

polysymptomatic hysteria, in which stress is expressed in a multiplicity of physical symptoms, and in which women predominate.

mass hysteria, in which members of a group, again mostly female, suffer from an outbreak of similar symptoms for which no physical explanation can be found.

Hysteria generally is said to be much rarer now than in the past and is believed to be yet another condition in which anxiety plays a precipitating role. Another explanation for its decline is that many illnesses formerly attributed to hysteria are now, thanks to the more sophisticated investigation techniques of modern medicine, diagnosed as having a physical cause.

In conversion hysteria (also called hysterical conversion), the apparent absence of anxiety, once a physical disability is established, is regarded as an important diagnostic sign. In contrast to the person who appears deeply concerned because of a real disability, the hysteric does not seem perturbed by his plight and exhibits the classic *belle indifference* which doctors look for when they suspect the presence of hysteria. The theory is that the patient unconsciously 'converts' emotions which he perceives as unacceptable and too difficult to explain into some more 'respectable' ailment which others are likely to find more acceptable. This may take the form of temporary blindness or paralysis or symptoms of a physical illness, for which no organic cause can be found. In another variant of conversion hysteria (called "dissociative hysteria"), the sufferer unconsciously blots out his memory of past events and develops an amnesia which cannot be explained. Experts suggest that in all these cases the patient is unconsciously motivated to seek escape from some difficult situation, such as a personal responsibility or stressful occupation, or some painful experience in the recent or more distant past. However, specialists stress the need for a thorough physical examination whenever conversion hysteria is suspected, and especially in those over 25 years old who develop such problems for the first time, so that some real organic ailment is not overlooked.

Once conversion hysteria is suspected and other tests

have proved negative, the GP usually refers the patient for psychiatric help. With reassurance, and, where possible, a reduction in the underlying stress factors, most sufferers regain their lost abilities fairly rapidly. Treatment may include behaviour therapy, hypnosis and sedative drugs. Where loss of memory is persistent, a form of therapy called 'abreaction' may be used by the psychiatrist: usually using hypnotherapy, the patient is helped to recall and discuss painful experiences which have been repressed, so that he can come to terms with them.

Polysymptomatic hysteria, a more common disorder, is thought to affect up to two per cent of women. In these cases, the patient visits the doctor very frequently over a long period because of numerous distressing physical complaints, many of them occurring simultaneously. These can include headache, dizziness, depression, muscular aches and pains, digestive disturbances, menstrual and sexual problems, urinary difficulties, visual disturbances. When numerous referrals to many different specialists produce no explanation for the patient's distress, her problem may be categorized as the 'fat file syndrome', a characteristic often shared by undiagnosed sufferers from severe anxiety and masked depression. With more insight into the patient's emotional problems, it may more accurately be labelled 'abnormal illness behaviour'.

Polysymptomatic hysteria (also known as Briquet's syndrome after the French doctor who described the condition in 1859) often starts in adolescence and continues indefinitely unless the problem is diagnosed and treated effectively. Instances of successful treatment were described by Cambridge consultant psychiatrist Dr A. R. K. Mitchell and Newmarket GP Dr I. R. Wallace in *The Practitioner* (May 1986). The approach they advocate requires the family doctor (with the participation of the family) to adopt a radically different attitude to the patient.

'He [the doctor] must stop looking at symptoms as a means of defining a physical diagnosis . . . He should consider the present symptoms as a kind of desperate communication: "I am unhappy with myself; I do not feel well; I do not think I can cope any longer with my life as it is;

I have come to see if you can help me." The patient's insistence on an organic pathology can be seen as a powerful need (usually successful) to engage the doctor's attention and then his care and concern, based on the assumption that emotional or psychological disorders are held by the medical profession, and society in general, to be of less importance than physical ones.'

Without challenging the patient's view of himself as a sick person, the doctor encourages him to discuss his perception of his overall situation, and the effect which his illness is having on him. The next step requires the doctor to ask, 'What help are you looking for?' This will often lead the doctor to reassess the patient's request for further investigations and to realize that the sufferer is distressed and is looking for helpful responses which have not yet been defined. The next step is for the doctor to establish a 'contract' with the patient, a mutually agreed bargain governing the time and duration of future interviews, and an understanding of the topics which will be discussed. Although some patients cannot cooperate in such a programme, many others can use it to gain a new lease of life free from the burden of chronic ill-health.

The most controversial form of hysteria is mass hysteria, an epidemic affliction in which numerous members of a group experience similar symptoms for which the cause is seen to be emotional rather than physical. Most of the victims are girls or young women who are supposed to be so 'suggestible' that once one of their number becomes dizzy or faints others rapidly follow her example.

While there seems to be little argument about mass hysteria being the explanation for some of these events, disagreements arise in relation to many others which might well be due to another cause. Modern authorities believe that the condition is much rarer than sensational reports of suspected episodes suggest; but when alternative explanations are forthcoming, these receive much less attention. For instance, when a large number of pupils in a girls' school were overcome by an illness thought to be mass hysteria some years ago, the event aroused widespread interest. When the real cause of the trouble was later shown to be toxic fumes which had somehow escaped into the classroom, the story was relegated to small print on inside pages.

One of the most famous outbreaks of suspected mass hysteria, in 1955, involved a very large number of mainly nursing staff at the Royal Free Hospital, London; it became known as 'Royal Free disease'. Another unexplained epidemic in 1970 affected nearly 150 nurses at Great Ormond Street's Hospital for Sick Children in London. Researchers found that both outbreaks had many features in common. Exhaustive laboratory investigations reported in the *British Medical Journal* (23 February 1974) pointed to an infection as the cause, but the researchers were unable to identify any infective source, such as a virus. Recently, however, the mystery appears to have been resolved. Research by leading London scientists, headed by Professor James Mowbray of St Mary's Hospital Medical School, has shown that a specific enterovirus (found in the intestines) is responsible for this type of outbreak. The illness it causes is called myalgic encephalomyelitis (ME), a lingering but non-fatal infection causing symptoms such as headache, poor concentration, extreme tiredness, digestive trouble, joint and muscle pain. Hailing the discovery as finally confirming his own long-held view, Dr Melvin Ramsay, president of the ME Association, who was in charge of the Royal Free Hospital's infectious diseases unit in 1955, said in a *Sunday Times* interview (25 January 1987): 'The medical profession was at fault because it swallowed the mass hysteria theory, hook, line and sinker. From the word go, some of us were certain that this was primarily a physical illness.' Now that a test is available to identify some forms of ME, at least one type of 'mass hysteria' appears to have become obsolete.

CHAPTER 5

Psychotic illness

Schizophrenia is the commonest psychotic disorder, affecting nearly one per cent of the population at some time in their lives. It is believed that, like many other illnesses, schizophrenia has a genetic component, which means that a predisposition to the disorder in the form of a subtle imbalance in body chemistry may be inherited.

It is also thought that even where a person is genetically vulnerable, the illness develops only where there is an additional environmental factor such as a virus to trigger an attack. The theory that a delayed-action virus may be responsible for the later onset of symptoms has gained support from the finding that sufferers are more likely to be born during the winter months, when the newborn baby is exposed to seasonal infections. This might also explain why most members of the sufferer's family remain free of the illness.

The name 'schizophrenia' derives from two Greek words meaning 'splitting of mind' and reflects the disturbances in thought and perception which are a characteristic of the illness. It is important not to confuse this term with the entirely unrelated concept of 'split mind' or 'split personality' as exemplified by the fictional Dr Jekyll and Mr Hyde, which is defined as a rare form of hysteria.

Because the illness varies with regard to the age at onset and the symptoms experienced by different patients, doctors often speak in terms of 'the schizophrenias' rather than of a single illness. In its most common and severe form it has its onset in the late teens or early twenties, and men tend to develop symptoms at an earlier age than women. A typical example is that of a hitherto bright and outgoing student who gradually loses the ability to concentrate, loses interest in friends and social activities, neglects his appearance, and becomes increasingly withdrawn from his family.

Such symptoms could be mistaken for a bad bout of severe depression, of course, and often are. But the diagnosis is seldom in doubt once the patient begins to display some of the more extreme changes in behaviour usually associated with schizophrenia. These can include feelings of persecution and the conviction that others are conspiring against him; listening to non-existent voices; being switched on to mysterious forces; imagining one's body is disintegrating and other delusions; rambling and incoherent speech and dramatic swings in mood.

On recovery, patients often can recall very clearly these acutely distressing periods. Explaining why she took an overdose, Wendy said: 'It seemed the only thing to do at the time. The voices were saying that I was a danger to my children and I had to protect them.' Dr Joyce Emerson wrote about a young man who believed his face was invisible, and had taken to wearing spectacles all the time so that he could be seen. An older man said he had 'dry rot of the bones, a kind of leprosy I picked up in Gibraltar.' A patient told Clare Marc Wallace: 'I just wanted to be away from people and listen to the voices. I hated my relatives for asking how I was. I often felt like smashing up the place. I wanted to die and used to think how I could do it.'

'About a third of sufferers experience only one episode; another third have further episodes with periods of remission in between; and the remainder experience the illness as a chronic condition they have to live with for the rest of their lives,' says MIND, the National Association for Mental Health. In the past, far fewer patients recovered sufficiently to lead normal lives, and a far greater number of those with chronic illness were destined to spend years in hospitals and other institutions. Credit for the dramatic turnaround in the control and prognosis of schizophrenia is attributed to the introduction of major tranquillizers in the early 1950s.

The most widely used group of major tranquillizers or anti-psychotic drugs are phenothiazines, which include Largactil, Melleril, Moditen, Modecate, Fentazin and

Stemetil. Depending on individual needs, these drugs are prescribed in syrup or tablet form, or as a weekly, fortnightly or monthly maintenance injection. Because withdrawal syndromes, though rare, can be severe, and the risk of relapse must always be borne in mind, withdrawal of anti-psychotic drugs should be undertaken only under the guidance of a specialist, according to the *Drug & Therapeutics Bulletin* (21 April 1987). Obviously, this advice is particularly important for patients who may be tempted to stop their medication without medical approval.

The most serious side-effect associated with the prolonged use of anti-psychotic drugs is tardive dyskinesia, a condition characterized by uncontrollable involuntary movements which affects between 15 and 20 per cent of patients. However, a report published in the *British Journal of Psychiatry* in 1986 suggests that susceptibility to this problem may be increased by advancing age and certain features of the underlying disease process in schizophrenia. Meanwhile, a new drug, known so far only as GR38032F and claimed to be more effective and to have far fewer side-effects than existing drugs, is being developed by Glaxo and Bradford University scientists. This is said to work by normalizing the production of dopamine, a brain control chemical which is understood to be overactive in schizophrenia.

Despite movements in the treatment of schizophrenia, severe hardship still tends to be the lot of a great many sufferers and their families. Not all patients discharged from hospital are well enough to survive in the community without adequate support, and many families find it impossible to cope with a difficult and disruptive son or daughter who still needs professional care in a residential setting. The trouble is that in many areas there is nowhere else the sick person can go, since the systematic reduction in mental hospital beds (including 30,000 beds lost in the six years up to the end of 1986) has never been matched by the promised alternative provision in the community for those needing it.

For as many as 8,000 mentally ill people with nowhere

else to go, prison represents the only sure source of food and shelter, a leading forensic psychiatrist told an experts' conference organized by the King Edward's Hospital Fund for London, early in 1987. In its evidence to a House of Commons committee in 1985, the British Medical Association estimated that less severely affected mentally abnormal offenders who should be receiving hospital care 'may constitute between 20 and 30 per cent of the sentenced population'. It seems ironic, to say the least, that the extent to which prisons have become a substitute for mental hospital accommodation is scarcely ever mentioned in the context of continuing concern about the very serious problem of overcrowding in prisons.

CHAPTER 6

The agony of anorexia nervosa

'I'm fully convinced that the biggest problem women have to contend with throughout their lives is a sense of inferiority in the first place because they are women, and secondly an inability to accept themselves as they really are at any given time,' says Judith, a former photographic model who believes she has finally reached a tranquil phase in her life after several years of intermittent hospital treatment for depression and eating problems.

'I think modelling is the most insecure career imaginable for a woman,' she explains. 'People envy you when they see you looking slim and beautiful and wearing fabulous clothes and probably earning quite a lot of money, but it's an extremely tough life and those who survive in it have to be very strong both emotionally and physically. When you get into it, as I did at seventeen, it's all so wonderful and you think you will go on for ever. Then you begin to realize that the price of continuing success is eternal vigilance, especially if you have an incipient weight problem, as I discovered I had. One day you look in the mirror and you realize that a pretty face and skinny figure are your sole assets, and without either nobody wants you. My way of dealing with the problem was to go overboard on exercise programmes and to cut down my diet to the point where I eventually became anorexic. And the joke was that everyone said I looked so good, and how did I manage it!

'In the end I got so depressed that I was bursting into tears at the most awkward moments and I couldn't go on working. My weight was down to six-and-a-half stone, which was very low for my height, and my periods had stopped altogether as they often do when someone is seriously under-weight. But my GP seemed to think there was nothing unusual about this when I went to ask him for something for my depression and sleep problems, though he seemed intrigued when I told him that I was a professional model. I've since heard that depression can be a symptom of anorexia, but I never met a doctor who commented on my low weight, although I saw several hospital specialists because of my depression and gynaecological problems over the next year or so. In fact, it was only when my mother got rather hysterical and rang up my GP that I was referred for treatment for anorexia. I really do think doctors could do a lot more to help women with eating problems, but I suspect they either don't notice the tell-tale signs or they fall into the trap of thinking that a slim figure adds up to health and beauty in a woman. I remember my mother's voice when she thought I couldn't hear her speaking to my GP on the telephone. "Can't you see she's a walking skeleton," she said. It was an exaggeration in my view, but perhaps not too much of an exaggeration.'

Judith was lucky in that she was among those sufferers from anorexia nervosa who can benefit from treatment in a hospital unit where the emphasis is on food intake and weight gain, combined with a behaviour therapy programme involving rewards for continuing progress. She attributes her relatively rapid recovery to the fact that her illness was due directly to the demands of her career, and that she had already begun to think along other lines by the time she was admitted to the special unit. 'It had been a slow and painful process and I didn't discuss it with anyone, but I was gradually becoming disenchanted with modelling, and had begun to think about finding some other kind of work.

'One day it came to me in a sort of blind flash that here I was at twenty-four with very little to show for my years of work, and that I wasn't qualified to do anything else. Eventually, I talked it over with my parents and I'm sure they thought it was a crazy idea when I said I wanted to go to university and read English. I had quite a few O-levels but not a single A-level at the time, so I had to start from scratch to qualify for entrance. But I made it and was accepted as a mature student and here I am! I don't think it would have been so easy for me if I hadn't had such supportive parents, or if I'd had some more serious psychological problems to account for my illness, as happens in many cases. I've no idea yet as to what I'll do with my degree when I get it. There are times when I still feel quite fragile emotionally, and I must confess that I haven't completely got over my obsession with food. But I think the advice I would give to anyone in my predicament is sound enough. I would say: Don't be afraid of change. If the job you're doing is making your life a misery, get out of it if you possibly can. And don't be misled into thinking that having a glamorous career is everything. For some of us it could even be a killer, as I nearly found out.'

In medical terms, anorexia simply means loss of appetite. The word is not strictly accurate in the case of anorexia nervosa, since the problem is not really loss of appetite but an irrational psychological fear of eating and of attaining normal body weight resulting in compulsive self-starvation. Though predominantly an illness of teenage girls, it does also affect younger children, boys and older women. It used to be thought that only about one boy was affected for every ten girls, but specialists now warn that the illness may be overlooked in boys and young men, and that the ratio of boys to girls may be much higher than previously suspected. Primary anorexia is defined as a phobia regarding weight, whereas the term secondary anorexia applies to the eating problem which develops when dieting to increase attractiveness gets out of control. Those who become anorectic in their twenties or thirties are more likely to be suffering from the secondary type.

A disturbing revelation of a growing trend towards anorexia among younger children, over a quarter of them boys, was made at the 1986 annual conference of the British Psychological Society in Sheffield. A study of 48 children aged between eight and fourteen, who between 1960 and 1984 were referred to Great Ormond Street Hospital for Sick Children, London, was described by Mrs Rachel Bryant-Waugh. The most common reason given by the children for refusing food was that they were 'afraid of becoming fat'. The majority came from homes in which there was open or repressed conflict between family members, and nearly half of those studied were the youngest children in the family, suggesting that over-protectiveness and early mealtime conflicts may have played a significant part in the development of the problem. In another report to the conference, Jane Wardle of the Institute of Psychiatry of London University described interviews with 348 children aged from twelve to eighteen who were pupils at a mixed-sex secondary school. All were of normal weight for age and height, yet three-quarters of the girls and just under two-fifths of the boys said they tried to control their weight by restricting their diet and by avoiding a wide range of nourishing foods as well as those with a high refined-carbohydrate content. Twelve-year-olds – especially the girls – were already markedly weight-conscious and concerned about their food intake.

Researchers studying anorexia describe it as a multifacto-rial disorder, one for which there is no adequate single explanation. Its traditional prevalence among teenage girls and young women led to the seemingly feasible suggestion that they used it as a means of rejecting sexual maturity and acquiring control over their own lives. Another finding is that anorectics come from families in which there are unstable relationships and communication is poor. Social pressures to conform to a fashionable ideal of slenderness obviously play an important role, as can belonging to a family in which there is an obsessive interest in food for one reason or another. The typical anorectic is seen as an otherwise healthy, intelligent and conscientious young person who often comes from a middle-class family.

Anorexia was recognized officially as a medical disorder about 1850, but one of the first descriptions of it on record was provided in the second century BC by Galen, one of the most influential doctors of Ancient Greece. In early Christian times fasting was seen as evidence of holiness and saintliness, according to modern medical historians. The legend of St Wilgefortis ('strong virgin'), who lived over a thousand years ago, was described in the *British Medical Journal* (18–25 December 1982) by an authority on eating problems, Dr J. Hubert Lacey of St George's Hospital, London.

St Wilgefortis was a daughter of the King of Portugal; having vowed to devote her life to God, she was distraught when her father arranged a marriage for her. She prayed earnestly for her beauty to be spoilt so that she would no longer be considered attractive, and God responded by causing hair to grow over her face and body. As a result, her suitor withdrew his proposal and her father had her put to death by crucifixion. The 'bearded saint', as she became known (female hirsutism due to hormone imbalance can be a complication of severe anorexia), attracted a large following among women in Europe in the succeeding centuries: a statue in her honour was erected in Henry VIII's Chapel in Westminster Abbey and another in Billingsgate, where she was known as 'St Uncumber' by women who sought her intercession so that they might be 'uncumbered' of troublesome husbands. 'What we now see as a disease produced by a complex inter-play of emotional, social, family, and existential dynamics, was viewed in pre-mediaeval Europe as a miracle: an attempt by minds unenlightened by the Renaissance to explain in a series of well-born girls an overwhelming fear of the implications of sexuality and marriage,' Dr Lacey concluded.

Supernatural influences were commonly believed in former times to be responsible for the phenomenon of 'fasting girls'. One of the most famous of these was a French girl, Jane Balan, whose story was recorded by Pedro Mexio in a book published in London in 1613. Her illness, which lasted for at least three years, began with fever and vomiting in her eleventh year, after which she refused food, 'for both meats and drinkes she altogether loaths and mightily abhorreth,' the author wrote.

Britain had its fair share of fasting girls too. The 'famed young Derbyshire damsel', Martha Taylor, was said to have lived for at least thirteen months with scarcely any food or drink, according to a 1669 report. Anne Moore, the 'fasting woman of Tutbury, Staffordshire', was believed to have survived without nourishment for six years beginning in 1807. However, she was one of the first to come under close medical observation, and it was noted that her weakened condition improved whenever surveillance was relaxed; she later admitted that she had taken some nourishment during her long fast.

A sadder fate awaited the 'Welsh fasting girl', Sarah Jacob. Sarah's illness began in 1867 when she was aged thirteen, and fell ill with pleurisy, fever and convulsions. She refused food for a month after her illness, made a brief recovery, and again resumed her fast, which continued intermittently until her death at the end of 1869. It was Sarah's misfortune that her fame as a 'miraculous faster' drew visitors from far and wide to her parents' isolated farmhouse in Carmarthenshire who 'were not discouraged from leaving monetary tokens'. She has been described as lying on a bed, prettily 'decorated as a bride, having around her head a wreath of flowers'.

'Sarah's reputation as a miraculous faster was seen as a matter of Welsh national honour and something that had to be defended against criticism by those who attacked what they regarded as local credulity and foolishness,' wrote Dr Gethin Morgan in the *British Medical Journal* (24–31 December 1977). To settle the question one way or the other, doctors decided on an experiment, which involved constant surveillance by a group of nurses, and strict monitoring of any food to which the child might have access. After eighteen days of this close watch, Sarah became seriously ill and died, apparently without anything being done to save her. Only the parents were punished for their part in the test, each receiving prison sentences with hard labour and losing their home. Yet, Dr Morgan speculates, Sarah might have succeeded in deceiving her parents so that they never realized she was eating secretly during the last two years of her life.

Although dating back well over a century, Sarah's case sheds light on one vital aspect of severe anorexia – the fact that the victim survives only because she is getting a little more nourishment than her family suspects. A characteristic which Sarah shared with most of today's anorectics and with Anne Moore was an obsessional reluctance to be seen to enjoy food, and a sense of guilt about taking nourishment. Because this rigid psychological barrier can be such a difficult one to penetrate, it goes without saying that too close observation other than in the structured environment of a special hospital unit may be self-defeating. Allowing the sufferer enough 'space' to break her self-imposed fast in private could be a life-saver.

Anorexia has been widely studied in recent years and, while it is claimed that its incidence has increased dramatically over the past two decades, it is also possible that some of this apparent increase is due both to greater awareness of the condition and to earlier medical consultation.

It is known that many anorectics start off with a moderate overweight problem, and may have been teased at school for this reason. Many have a perfectionist streak and a horror of failure, so their illness may be triggered by disappointing exam results. Others starve themselves to punish their bodies because of feelings of guilt and self-hatred. Often the sufferer's family is one in which emotions are suppressed, and there is little communication about matters of personal importance to individual members. Inadequately expressed grief is a modern phenomenon which can lead to lasting emotional problems and can also be a root cause of anorexia, as Dr Robert McAll, a British doctor, showed in a letter to *The Lancet* in 1980. He found that in fifteen cases of anorexia which he treated, a member of the family had died without being properly mourned. One girl weighing only five-and-a-half stone, and for whom hospital treatment had been unsuccessful, needed to mourn for her father who had been killed in a car accident when she was eleven; a middle-aged man who had been anorectic for over twenty years had felt guilty about persuading his wife to have an abortion before they were married. Once patients were provided with a 'means of repentance' through participation in a church service of mourning, dramatic improvements were achieved, Dr McAll reported.

As in the case of St Wilgefortis who died to preserve her virginity over a thousand years ago, rejection of developing sexuality and its broader implications continues to be regarded as a contributing factor in anorexia among women. One recovered anorectic – a woman doctor – described her own experience some years ago: 'The fact that many cases of anorexia seem to occur between the ages of fifteen and eighteen shows that sexual awareness plays an important part. Exactly what type of sexual awareness is an individual matter. At the time of my illness the permissive age was just starting and I remember feeling both sickened and horrified by the growing emphasis placed on man's gross appetites . . . My protest was against the moral decline around me, but the only way I could protest was to deprive myself of the most basic need – food. By a decreased intake of food, the natural process of physical development was staved off, and I was prolonging the protection of a familiar and pleasanter stage – childhood. Rather like the nun who denies herself everything and enters an enclosed order, the anorectic has taken upon herself the burden of purging the world in the only way she, in her immaturity, knows how.' (*British Medical Journal*, 24 June 1978).

It is estimated that about five per cent of anorectics die within five years; in such cases the most common cause of death is suicide due to the depression usually associated with the condition. A more positive way of regarding this statistic is to remember that 95 out of every 100 people affected do eventually recover. Sometimes recovery takes place seemingly spontaneously after some years, perhaps because the sufferer has developed a more mature outlook on life. Another explanation may be that she has come to terms with the emotional problems which gave rise to anorexia in the first place.

The treatment of anorexia is very often a slow process calling for patience, hope and determination on the part of everyone concerned. Convincing the patient that she needs help and obtaining her cooperation can be crucial in cutting short the duration of the illness in the early stages. In cases of severe weight loss, hospital treatment is essential. As the condition becomes better understood, more effective strategies are being developed with the aim of encouraging the patient to change her attitude to food and to increase her weight. In some programmes the emphasis is on weight gain, with rewards – such as visits from relatives – being offered as an inducement; while behaviour therapy of this kind may seem harsh, it is reported to be very successful with many patients. For those who are very ill and are still resistant to treatment, more intensive medical and nursing care is needed. Sedative drugs and psychotherapy are often used to help break down resistance to nutrition.

Once 80 per cent of the normal weight has been regained there usually is a marked improvement in the patient's psychological outlook, according to Dr Peter Dally and Dr Joan Gomez, authors of a study on the subject. But, they insist, progress in severe cases needs to be measured in years rather than months. On the brighter side, they found that girls with mild anorexia which had lasted for less than a year usually made a rapid recovery without hospitalization once their problem had been recognized. At the end of two years, 38 per cent of all their patients had reached 90 per cent or more of their original weight, and the proportion achieving this level of success had almost doubled in four years.

Studies of family relationships have tended to discount the earlier theory that mothers of anorectics were likely to be inordinately dominant and over-protective towards the ill child before the illness. Dr Dally and Dr Gomez found that, on the whole, anorectics came from relatively stable families, though younger teenagers were more likely to have depressed mothers. A quarter of their patients came from homes in which there were 'unusually strong eating eccentricities', with special emphasis being placed on vegetarian and 'natural' foods or on the avoidance of certain items, such as red meat or animal fats. In common with other recent studies, they found a comparatively high tendency for anorexia and other eating disorders to affect more than one member of the family, adding that anorexia and hysteria can reach epidemic proportions in girls' boarding schools, following the example of a 'ringleader'.

One point on which doctors and patients usually agree is that, rightly or wrongly, the anorectic sees herself as being overweight. Even when she has lost a great deal of weight and is quite emaciated, she still complains that she is too fat and worries about getting fatter. It is this typical distortion of the 'self-image' which makes it so difficult for her to admit that she is ill and needs treatment: 'Although my clothes were literally falling off me, and I was buying clothes two, then three, then four sizes smaller, I sincerely believed that the clothes I had had simply stretched.' Thus did a member of the self-help group Anorexic Aid describe her own four-year ordeal.

It was only on admission to hospital weighing less than five stone that Renée Kauffer finally accepted that she was suffering from anorexia. Then, in order to be able to accept treatment and start eating again, she had to contend with another crucial psychological barrier, the loss of personal control over her own food intake, weight and lifestyle. 'These feelings of control grow stronger and stronger as all else in your little world seems to be crumbling. There is even great satisfaction in the gnawing hunger pains, because they prove that you haven't eaten too much.'

In reality, the sense of 'being in control', which is common to anorectics, is symbolic of increasing autonomy over only one facet of existence, combined with loss of control over life in general: 'At five-and-a-half stone and under, you literally cannot think. You block out all of your emotions. You concentrate on limiting your nutritional intake to something like 80 calories a day, and you go through the whole day worrying about how you are going to remain within this limit,' Professor Arthur Crisp of St George's Hospital, London, explained in a recent BBC Radio 4 phone-in programme. He sees teenage anorexia as a 'coping mechanism' used, in much the same way that others use alcohol, to deal with the stresses and psychological problems commonly associated with puberty and the inescapable transition from childhood to adult status. The onset of teenage anorexia often coincides with other problems at home and at school, such as the break-up of the parents' marriage, anxiety about exams, financial worries in the family, and feelings of rejection resulting from the failure of a teenage romance.

However, it is unfair to blame families – or for families to blame themselves – when a teenager becomes anorectic or resorts to anti-social behaviour of some other kind, such as drug abuse. Since members of the caring professions seldom know a family intimately enough to pass judgement before a problem arises affecting one member, they have difficulty in establishing which came first – the over-anxious and excessively protective mother or the child's illness. Was the father always as tetchy and uncommunicative as he has become of late? Were the brothers and sisters always as competitive and self-centred as they now appear to be, or have they become that way in a desperate battle for parental attention in a home where so much care is focused on the sick member of the family? Did the husband and wife always blame each other when things went wrong, or has this pattern of behaviour developed only since the child became ill?

Rita, whose daughter Barbara was anorectic for five years and has now recovered, says the comparison is a fair one only to a limited extent. 'Over the years, there was nothing about Barbara's early development to suggest that she would have this terrible problem, which started when she was fourteen. If it was due to something we did wrong, then why weren't her brother and sister also affected? This is a question we asked ourselves over and over again in the early stages. There were differences in their personalities, we could see. We thought it was something to do with being the eldest that made her more nervy and anxious than the younger ones, who were a very happy-go-lucky pair. She used to worry a lot about her schoolwork and about being punctual, for example.

'We had no idea that there was anything wrong with Barbara, until one day I happened to go into her bedroom while she was dressing and saw how painfully thin she was. You could count her ribs, as they say. I just stood there unable to speak, and she was furiously indignant about her privacy being invaded. On reflection, I realized that I hadn't noticed her thinness because she always wore loose clothes, such as chunky sweaters, track-suits and the like. I also began to think about her eating habits, and all the

115

times she wouldn't eat with the family, because she'd eaten at school or at a friend's house, or was rushed for time and would have a snack somewhere. The fact of the matter was that she wasn't eating anywhere most of the time, except for the occasional cup of black coffee and dry cream cracker she would allow herself at home.

'We did have enough authority over Barbara to get her to see the doctor under protest that we were making a fuss about nothing. Twice, when her weight was down to around five stone, we got her into hospital, but she wouldn't cooperate. We paid for her to have private psychotherapy for over a year but, in the end, the therapist didn't want to continue because he felt we were wasting money. Then, one day, when we had more or less given up hope, she suddenly started eating again – just a little at first but it was a beginning, and she never looked back. It had been a dreadful five years for our family, and the younger ones suffered neglect.

'We could never take a holiday, for instance. They were always complaining about Barbara, insisting that she was selfish and self-centred, which she was; and I found their behaviour an additional worry as they got older, but they eventually settled down, I'm happy to say. Then there was a stage when my husband said it was all too much for him, and he left home for about six months. I can't say I blamed him. There were times when I wished that I could get away. I couldn't see any way out. I still see Barbara's recovery as nothing short of a miracle, and it is only now after two years that I'm beginning to stop worrying.'

BULIMIA NERVOSA
It is estimated that about one-third of anorectics at low body weight resort to bingeing and self-induced vomiting afterwards as a method of meeting their craving for energy foods without gaining weight. This condition has existed for a long time, although it has come to public attention only in recent years. In addition, many anorectics also take large doses of laxatives with the aim of preventing the absorption of nutrients in the digestive tract from the small amount of food they do manage to swallow. Both of these

practices are difficult to detect because they are carried out secretly, and both can cause serious damage to health.

Relatively little was known about bulimia and the extent of its use among women until research psychiatrist Dr Christopher Fairburn placed a notice in the magazine *Cosmopolitan* in 1980, inviting women with experience of the condition to complete a confidential questionnaire. He received 620 replies, of which 83 per cent supplied information consistent with a diagnosis of bulimia nervosa. Over 56 per cent said they induced vomiting at least once daily. Most were of normal weight, but over 68 per cent showed pronounced signs of emotional illness, and 89 per cent had 'profoundly disturbed attitudes to food and eating'. Over 56 per cent thought they needed medical help, but only 30 per cent had discussed their eating problems with a doctor. Less than half of the women reported having had anorexia in the past. The average duration of the problem was four-and-a-half years. It is well known that when weight drops below a certain level, either through starvation or too strenuous exercise, menstruation ceases and women become infertile temporarily until weight is restored. Almost half of these women ex- perienced menstrual irregularity, suggesting that abnormal eating habits may interfere with the menstrual cycle, irrespec- tive of body weight (*British Medical Journal*, 17 April 1982).

The most famous self-confessed victim of bulimia is undoubtedly the American film actress, Jane Fonda, who decided when she was in her mid-forties to tell the world about her 23-year battle against the disorder. Her nightmare began when she was twelve years old and in boarding school, at a time when she enjoyed eating but wanted to be slim: 'It didn't take long for me to become a bulimic – bingeing and purging 15 to 20 times a day. I would literally empty a refrigerator. It's an addiction like drugs or alcohol.' Jane Fonda was thirty-five by the time she kicked the bulimic habit, after a lifetime of agony when she couldn't admit even to herself that she suffered from a serious illness so out of keeping with her public image as a supremely self-confident achiever. Another brilliant, self-assertive American woman who finally won her own

20-year battle against anorexia and bulimia is Kim Chernin, poet, fiction writer and psychotherapist. Both women express serious concern about contemporary trends in the United States, where up to 30 per cent of women – and perhaps a higher proportion of students – suffer from the disorder.

A survey of 1,728 American teenagers carried out at Stanford University and reported in 1986 in the *Journal of the American Medical Association* found that 13 per cent engaged in regular purging as a means of weight control. Of these, two-thirds were girls and one-third were boys. 'Both male and female purgers felt more guilty after eating large amounts of food, counted calories more often, dieted more frequently, and exercised less than non-purgers.' Binge-eating followed by laxative abuse and self-induced vomiting has become a widespread practice in the United States, where doctors are constantly stressing its dangers to physical and emotional health.

What causes some people – predominantly women – to resort to bulimia in the first place, and then to become enslaved to binge-eating and vomiting for years on end? For the most part, bulimia is regarded as a behavioural disorder usually associated with stress within the family and in other relationships. Doctors have pointed out that, very occasionally, compulsive over-eating may be due to some physical problem, the most likely being some imbalance affecting the appetite control centre in the brain. Laboratory studies aimed at discovering some chemical imbalance which might provide a key to the condition (such as those carried out at Stanford University) have found few blood abnormalities among those investigated.

Various theories have been put forward to explain the psychological roots of the disorder. Susie Orbach attributes eating problems to cultural conditioning: the message coming clearly to women from advertising and women's magazines is 'diet, deprive and deny'; food is no longer a basic essential and something to be enjoyed heartily – it is the enemy which must be brought under control at all costs. She also sees maternal attitudes to the development of daughters, and an ambivalent 'push-pull dynamic in the mother-daughter relationship', providing encouragement on the one hand, imposing restraints and thwarting initiative on the other, as important contributing factors. Mothers traditionally take pride in their sons' healthy appetites, but hover anxiously over their daughters' food preferences, she argues. In her own successful therapy programme for eating disorders, psychotherapy is structured towards unravelling underlying conflicts and working through painful feelings associated with the disorder.

As so many sufferers have testified, the life of a bulimic is a profoundly unhappy and guilt-ridden one. In a study among young American women, Dr Sandra Weiss of the United States National Institute of Mental Health found a high rate of psychological problems and impulsive behaviour tendencies among sufferers. Those participating complained of severe depression, anxiety, poor self-esteem, and difficulties with personal relationships. They felt they lacked control over their own lives. Some indulged in binge-buying, theft and drug-abuse; and some of them had attempted suicide.

Although bulimics are often found to be of normal weight, their illness can have numerous adverse effects on their physical health, some of them very serious. Symptoms of indigestion, such as heartburn, are common. Persistent vomiting can cause damage to the enamel of the teeth, chronic irritation of the mouth cavity, painful enlargement of the salivary glands, oedema (water retention in the tissues) and 'bloating'. More serious complications include abnormal dilation of the stomach, tearing of the gullet and kidney failure.

Another risk, which has been recognized only in recent years, is that chronic anorexia and bulimia may – in certain cases – lead to premature loss of bone substance (osteoporosis), a condition usually seen only in some older women after the menopause, which can increase the risk of fractures. This has been found to occur in women with a long-term history of absent periods, the explanation being that very low weight and under-nutrition causes depletion of natural oestrogen in the body. Very thin vegetarian women who avoid milk as well as meat (dietary sources of oestrogen) are especially at risk, Professor Howard Jacobs, head of the department of reproductive endocrinology at the Middlesex Hospital, London, told a recent medical conference. This discovery is yet one more compelling reason for women with eating problems to seek medical advice promptly.

For anyone with a serious eating problem, the first person to see is the family doctor, who will be able to arrange a referral to a specialist if necessary, and to advise about local self-help and therapy groups. While seriously ill patients still need hospital treatment (and in extreme cases can be admitted to hospital under the Mental Health Act if they refuse treatment), very successful programmes have been developed to provide therapy on an out-patient basis.

The ideal approach to eating problems would be to catch them in the incipient stages before they become an established practice. Obviously, this is not an easy matter, since research has shown that too much concentration on food in a household may contribute to the development of anorexia, and paying too much attention to the eating habits of someone in the family (toddlers as well as teenagers and young adults) can lead to resistance and a battle of wits, which, in the case of a potential anorectic, may result in furtive food avoidance. Another difficulty is that an eating problem may already be well established by the time there is any noticeable weight loss, and even then loose garments, much favoured by many anorectics, can be misleading. Persuading a teenager or young adult to see the doctor and to discuss eating problems is a task calling for tact and patience and a discreet advance warning to the doctor in case the patient evades the basic issue, which often happens.

A screening test to identify the *potential* anorectic has been designed by clinical psychologist Dr Peter Slade of Liverpool University, according to a *Sunday Times* report by Helen Mason (7 December 1986). His finding is that those who are susceptible tend to display two key personality characteristics: *perfectionism* (a trait which parents and teachers tend to encourage, but which, taken to extremes, involves setting unattainable standards and profound dissatisfaction with every aspect of life); and the feeling of *not being in control* which results from failure in perfectionism (self-starvation and weight loss give the anorectic a false sense of control).

Once these risk factors have been identified, the next step is very forthright preventive counselling, which works well according to the Liverpool team's experience. 'I put the fear of God into them,' Dr Slade says. 'I describe the course they are actually embarked on, and all the problems they are going to go through.' This means spelling out in very clear language the mental and physical horrors associated with anorexia. Let us hope that the National Health Service will take notice.

In the meantime, one thing we should all aim for is a healthier attitude to food generally. Instead of the confusion existing at present with regard to a huge range of real or imaginary risks claimed to be involved in food production and processing, let us have some common-sense guidance, and a more critical assessment of some of the food advertisements seen on television screens at peak viewing times for young people.

Kim Chernin sees the alarming rise in the incidence of eating problems among American women as a direct offshoot of the feminist movement. She argues that men have responded to the threat which its liberating influence has posed for them, and to evidence of growing feminine power, by stepping up their efforts to promote the unrealistic ideal of the ultra-slender 'child-woman' who is easier to control. Girls are falling into the trap at an increasingly earlier age and reacting to this all-pervasive conditioning by becoming obsessed with body weight, food and food-avoidance. In this she sees a parallel between women's suffrage early in the twentieth century and the cult of boyish slimness which subsequently developed in the 1920s and later. A dramatic revolution in the type of clothes worn by women certainly took place after World War I, brought on by practical considerations. Gone forever (and good riddance) were the voluminous under-garments, thickly gathered at the waist and flounced to the ground; gone were the concealing outer garments. All right, said the men, buxom wenches are out. Suddenly, women couldn't afford not to worry about their circumference and their food intake, and so it has been ever since. Insofar as powerful men ruled and still rule the world of women's fashions and advertising, Kim Chernin's argument is indeed a persuasive one. The vogue took off in real earnest with the demands of the American film industry, and in the 1960s everyone wanted to look like Twiggy, the skinny model who became an international star. Doctors could only complain increasingly as they watched the soaring incidence of anorexia among young women.

Now that we are into the late 1980s, and Twiggy has been transformed into a beautiful woman with nicely rounded contours, is there a chance that the mighty ones who so successfully manipulate women through the medium of fashion might be about to allow them a little more latitude? According to *Observer Magazine* writer, Veronica Horwell (7 December 1986), the indications are promising. Lean times have gone and 'big girls' are coming into their own. 'There haven't been so many substantial women around since the Edwardian era, when the goddesses were 6ft, size 16 . . . and ripeness was all.' But, even so, 'The bust has never been readmitted to couture. Dior's New Look of 1947 is always billed as the most feminine line, but the models who wore it were size 10 maximum, just corseted and padded subtly to suggest curves, while their faces and limbs remained stick-frail.' In a recent exploration of the Yves St Laurent fashion museum in Paris (covering 30 years in time and five floors in space), Ms Horwell failed to find even one garment designed for a hip measuring more than 36 inches. 'As designers were increasingly attracted to the perfect blank bodyscreen of pre-pubescent girls, adult women pursued a biological impossibility – to be undernourished but healthy, and aged thirteen for life.' Then, about two years ago, Ms Horwell noticed some welcome changes. Designers began displaying their clothes on women with 37in busts, larger ladies were being chosen for romantic film roles and curves seemed to be on the way in again. Let us hope that the trend lasts long enough to counteract the pernicious conditioning of the past 70 years.

While there clearly are emotional and psychological factors involved, both in the initiation of eating problems, and their continuance once anorexia or bulimia has taken root as a way of life, and while fashion trends obviously play a crucial role, example can also be a potent influence. In a 1985 report in the *British Journal of Psychiatry*, the pattern of one 17-year-old girl's progression was described by a team at the Maudsley Hospital, London. Their patient was an apparently healthy student when she made friends with four other students – tall, slim girls who worked part-time as models. Soon she was joining them at their weekly tea party, where they all feasted on fattening carbohydrate foods like cakes and doughnuts. Then, their appetites sated, they would retire to the bathroom in turn to make themselves vomit. Predictably, this routine eventually led to trouble. Four of the five girls developed anorexia, and two of them became so ill that they needed to be admitted to hospital.

An interesting observation made by several researchers is that most anorexics and bulimics tend to be exceptionally good-looking, despite dissatisfaction with personal appearance being such a common feature of both conditions. Could it be that good looks in themselves tend to predispose to eating disorders, insofar as physical beauty may heighten self-awareness in a negative sense, leading to inordinate anxiety regarding its preservation? Or, in view of the prevalence of these problems among models, actresses and dancers, might not the explanation be that attractive girls are encouraged to choose careers which are by their nature insecure, often limited in tenure, and dependent on the retention of a slender figure and youthful good looks? Perhaps it would help if all young girls were encouraged to train for long-term employment, even if their sights were set on a more glamorous career in the short term.

CHAPTER 7

Women and wine

'Good wine is a good familiar creature if it be well used,' wrote Shakespeare in *Othello*; much earlier, an Old Testament philosopher spoke warmly of the 'wine that maketh glad the heart of man.' In song and story down the ages, drink has more often been extolled as a worthy friend than blamed as a treacherous enemy, and so it is seen largely up to the present time, despite ample evidence of the ravages which excessive indulgence can create for the unwary.

Like much else that women were not supposed to enjoy in times past, drink was traditionally a male preserve. 'Man, being reasonable, must get drunk,' observed Byron; and society has always been tolerant towards the occasional lapse from sobriety on the part of its menfolk. But the best a woman with a similar weakness might hope for was a disreputable perch beside the Sarah Gamps and other gin-swilling harridans of English literature. So, inevitably, the history of alcohol enjoyment among women is one of demeaning secrecy, furtive tippling, and mysterious female maladies for which humiliating allowances had to be made. Small wonder that so many 'respectable ladies' reached gratefully for that most euphemistic of Victorian inventions, 'invalid wine', like Aunt Pittypat's 'swoon bottle' in *Gone With the Wind*.

All that has changed dramatically. Drinking for women finally became acceptable, not through any effort of the women's movement, but as a result of commercial expedience: twice as many drinkers means twice as much profit. Between them, drink manufacturers spend more than £100 million a year on advertising, according to the Health Education Council which, before its recent replacement by the new Health Education Authority, campaigned strenuously against smoking and alcohol abuse for many years. The Council cites the case of one company which recently invested £5 million in a cinema advertising campaign aimed at a largely teenage audience. Nor is there much incentive for the Government to back an effective campaign against alcohol abuse, since the Exchequer benefits from taxes on alcohol to the tune of £6,000 million a year, or £11,000 every minute.

Even more insidious than advertising is the manner in which drink is promoted through feature programmes on television. In episode after episode, American 'soap operas' drive home the message that a regular intake of strong liquor is an essential prerequisite of the glamorous life, *Dallas* or *Dynasty* style. As JR reaches once again for the whisky decanter, as Alexis sips from a sparkling glass for the umpteenth time, the connection is unmistakable: alcohol is the fuel which keeps these two powerful characters firing on all cylinders. We have our own home-grown examples, of course, and not only on television. In the long-running radio saga of farming folk, *The Archers*, most of the action worth noting revolves round the pub or the wine bar. In neither venue is there ever a suggestion of rowdiness or even of 'tired and emotional' behaviour on the part of the 'locals'. Nobody gets drunk, nobody develops cirrhosis, and we are left in no doubt that Elizabeth, the trendy teenage daughter of Ambridge's first family and the only one who has any real fun, has been thriving on a regular diet of gin-and-tonic from an early age.

In real life the picture is seldom so cosy. Approximately one million people experience serious drink problems in the United Kingdom. According to Professor John Strong, first chairman of Action on Alcohol Abuse (AAA or 'Triple A'), the new campaigning organisation established in 1983 by the Conference of Medical Royal Colleges in Britain, 'Alcohol abuse affects far more than the individual primarily involved. We are all to some extent at risk.' One-third of all divorce petitions cite alcohol as a contributory factor. One-third of all child abuse cases are linked to regular heavy use of alcohol by a parent.

Alcohol-induced sickness is responsible for the loss to industry of over eight million working days each year. Alcohol intoxication is involved in the deaths of over 500 young people each year – up to 10 per cent of all deaths in persons under 25 – and over 50 per cent of homicides (with nearly 50 per cent of the victims also being intoxicated).'

While the great majority of heavy drinkers are still men, recent statistics show that the rates for women have been rising more rapidly than those for men with regard to convictions for drunkenness and drunken driving, mental hospital admissions due to alcohol abuse, and deaths from cirrhosis of the liver. The growing number of women with serious health and social problems has been causing concern for many years and, because these so often result in anxiety and depression for which alcohol is promoted as a form of relief, it is important to understand as much as possible about its effects.

The Royal College of Psychiatrists' 1979 report says it is a matter of the utmost importance to understand the social processes that can play a part in the genesis of alcoholism. 'What can be asserted is that if the average man or woman begins to drink more, then the number of people who damage themselves by their drinking will also increase. "Normal drinking" and excessive drinking are not two distinct species of behaviour with entirely different determinants . . . This statement runs contrary to the comfortable and previously accepted view that alcoholism is a disease from which a minority of unfortunate people are destined to suffer, whatever the general availability of alcohol.'

Doctors who specialize in this field consider it important to distinguish between heavy drinkers for whom alcohol abuse is a primary problem, and those who use alcohol predominantly to suppress symptoms of depression or anxiety but to an extent where it becomes a problem in its own right – a secondary problem. In the latter case, discovering and treating the underlying cause increase the chance of rapid recovery from the drink problem, as was found in one three-year follow-up study of women with secondary alcoholism who were given anti-depressants for primary depression. In other words, depression usually is easier to treat than a socially-motivated drinking problem. However, once drinking gets out of hand, it is seldom easy to see the problem as anything but a drink problem.

By virtue of the nature of their work, commercial travellers, barmen, journalists and workers in the building trade are more likely to get into regular drinking habits than those following a more conventional routine. For young people working away from home or lacking social facilities in their own environment, the pub is often the only outlet offering escape from loneliness. If they are unlucky, they more or less drift into a pattern of heavy drinking which eventually gets out of control, leaving no room in their lives for more rewarding activities. Yet remembering how drinking began can be crucial when it comes to seeking help.

In one of the first studies of its kind, researchers at King's College Hospital's Liver Unit found that a high proportion of 71 patients with alcoholic liver disease had suffered from psychiatric illnesses before developing drink problems (*British Medical Journal*, 12 November 1983). Of these, the most common conditions included depression and anxiety. It is a sobering thought that timely treatment for these symptoms might have cut short the drink problems in some cases and prevented the development of a potentially serious illness. Clearly, there is a strong case for seeking medical help for alcohol problems in the early stages, when underlying emotional illness can be more easily diagnosed and treated.

HOW ALCOHOL INTAKE IS MEASURED
Because it is vital for us to know the limits which are considered safe from a health point of view and how to check our consumption on a daily or weekly basis, alcohol values have been standardized in a way that is easier to understand. The agreed measure used for this purpose is the *standard unit*.

One standard unit is equal to one centilitre of alcohol in volume or approximately 10 grams in weight. This is the equivalent of one small glass of sherry; one glass of table wine; one single measure of whisky; half a pint of ordinary beer or cider; one-third pint of strong beer. Measures used in the home are likely to be over-generous. Calculated by the bottle, one litre bottle of table wine contains 10 units; one bottle of sherry 12 units; one bottle of spirits 30 units; a quart bottle of average cider 6 units; a quart of strong cider 8 units.

We are reminded by the Transport and Road Research Laboratory in its literature that the standard unit applies to *English measures*: Scottish spirit measures are 20 per cent greater than English ones, and spirit measures in Northern Ireland are 50 per cent greater.

HOW MUCH ALCOHOL IS SAFE FOR HEALTH?

Because individual men and women differ in the way their bodies deal with alcohol, no one claims to have established the definitive answer to this question for everyone. What is certain is that earlier estimates of maximum safety levels are now considered excessive, on the basis of more recent research. Four major reports published in 1986 from the Royal Colleges of Physicians, Psychiatrists and General Practitioners, and the British Psychological Society, have led to an agreed table of limits which is being publicized by Alcohol Concern.

The new limits, above which possible damage to health may occur, are 21 units a week for women and 35 units a week for men. For the least risk, women should confine themselves to 14 units and men to 21 units per week. Anyone currently exceeding these upper safety limits of 21 and 35 units (and 3 per cent of women and 14 per cent of men do) are advised to reduce their drinking immediately.

WHY WOMEN ARE MORE VULNERABLE

The main explanation for the greater risks to women from alcohol relates to body size and differences between the sexes in the distribution of fatty tissue and water. On average, women are lighter in weight than men but, when compared with men of equal weight, women are still at a disadvantage. When alcohol is absorbed into the bloodstream and is distributed throughout the body, it mixes evenly with the water which makes up nearly two-thirds of body weight. Because women's bodies contain less water, and proportionately more fatty tissue, alcohol consumed has to circulate in a smaller volume of fluid. This is reflected in a higher blood alcohol level than that of a man consuming an equal amount of alcohol over the same period. It follows that a woman will reach the legal limit for motor drivers more quickly and become inebriated more rapidly than her male counterpart.

Blood alcohol levels are expressed in terms of milligrams (mg) of alcohol per 100 millilitres (ml) of blood. In Britain, the legal limit for motor drivers is 80mg/100ml of blood, and 107mg/100ml of urine. The limit for the smaller amount of alcohol in the breath is 35 micrograms/100ml.

In theory, an 11-stone man drinking one pint of beer (two units of alcohol) quickly on an empty stomach will have a blood alcohol level 'peaking' at 30mg/100ml after about one hour; if he takes no further drink, the level will fall at the rate of approximately one unit per hour. However, because absorption rates vary so much, it is never possible to forecast blood alcohol levels reliably on the basis of intake, according to the Transport and Road Research Laboratory in Berkshire. What is easier to measure is the rate at which alcohol is excreted from the body, which *is* one unit per hour. Another important way in which women are at a disadvantage is in the smaller size of the female liver, the organ which has the task of processing alcohol, changing it chemically so that toxic products do not accumulate and facilitating its eventual removal from the body. Thus, elimination of alcohol occurs more slowly in women, another reason for disproportionately higher blood alcohol levels than for men with an equal consumption. Much more serious, however, is the far greater risk of liver disease, even for women who are relatively moderate drinkers. Between 1979 and 1984, deaths from liver cirrhosis among women increased by 65 per cent compared with a 46 per cent increase for men, who, in numerical terms, still form the majority of heavy drinkers.

A report on research findings at King's College
Hospital's Liver Unit by writer Brigid McConville shows
that 40 per cent of current cirrhosis patients are women,
and that it is possible for them to develop the disease on a
regular intake of 40 grams of alcohol a day or even less (four
units – four glasses of table wine or four small whiskies).
Other factors found to increase women's vulnerability to
alcohol include the contraceptive pill (which slows down
the metabolism of alcohol), biological changes such as
ovulation (midway between periods), and the premenstrual phase in the menstrual cycle.

More than any other organ in the body, the liver is at risk
from heavy drinking because of its major role in processing
alcohol, and because of the way in which this increased
work-load can interfere with its routine responsibilities:
storage of sugar, processing of fats, secretion of bile, and
many other important functions.

The liver's susceptibility to damage is so widely
recognized that the risk of cirrhosis is something which
worries most heavy drinkers from time to time.
Unfortunately too many adopt a fatalistic attitude in the
belief that irretrievable harm has already been done, and
continue drinking. Yet, even where damage has been
confirmed through medical investigation, cirrhosis need
not be a death sentence, provided that the sufferer stops
drinking, the Royal College of Psychiatrists says in its 1979
report. 'The important message for the patient with
alcohol-induced liver disease is that, if he goes on drinking,
his liver condition will further deteriorate, with cirrhosis
meaning an extremely unpleasant form of invalidism and a
much curtailed life expectancy. Emphasis must also be
placed on the fact that, if the patient stops drinking, the
liver disease will often cease to progress. There are few
circumstances in which abstinence can be so life-saving.'

Both men and women, even if only moderate drinkers,
can suffer from milder forms of liver damage, such as
alcoholic hepatitis (inflammation) and enlargement due to
fatty infiltration, conditions which if drinking continues
can lead in time to cirrhosis. The average liver can cope
pretty well with reasonable amounts of alcohol, but when

an excessive ingestion of alcohol forces it to overwork, it cannot keep up with its other urgent tasks. Fats are allowed to accumulate, leading to the problem of 'fatty liver' and chronic enlargement, and the release of sugar into the bloodstream may be too slow to maintain normal blood sugar levels. Reactive hypoglycaemia (low blood sugar) can also affect vulnerable individuals who drink on an empty stomach, causing symptoms such as weakness, dizziness, irritability and even mental confusion (which may be mistaken for drunkenness) two or three hours later. Since severe hypoglycaemia can lead to coma, it is worth remembering that a cup of sweet tea or coffee helps to restore the balance in such cases.

It is always wise to ask the doctor if alcohol is safe to take when a drug is being prescribed. As a depressant drug which achieves its 'high' by damping down certain activity in the brain, alcohol can be dangerous if combined with other drugs which depress brain function, including anti-depressants, tranquillizers, barbiturates (now strictly controlled because of their increased risks) and, of course, opiates such as heroin. Milder preparations whose sedative effects can be enhanced by alcohol include antihistamines, anti-travel sickness pills, and pain-killers obtainable without prescription.

A variety of other drugs may cause problems, producing toxic effects, having their action enhanced, or requiring caution because of a possible interaction with alcohol, according to *Drug Interaction Alert* (Boehringer Ingelheim). For instance a potentially serious toxic reaction may occur if anti-diabetic preparations containing chlorpropamide are combined with alcohol. Caution is also advised with regard to alcohol consumption for patients being prescribed metronidazole, a treatment commonly used for trichomonal vaginal infection (trade names include Flagyl).

It is estimated that one man in every five admitted to hospital in Britain is suffering from an alcohol-related illness, but the proportion may be higher than this in many areas. In a study at St Charles' Hospital in west London, it was found that over a quarter of 104 men and women patients admitted for emergency treatment were suffering from alcohol-related conditions (*Journal of the Royal Society of Medicine*, March 1986): 28 per cent of men and 20 per cent of women had drunk more than the equivalent of 20 measures of spirits or 10 pints of beer in the previous week. The reasons for admission included deliberate drug overdoses in nine cases, severe chest infections, psychological difficulties related to drinking, and complaints which were thought to have arisen largely through self-neglect. A detailed inquiry into the drinking habits of all acutely ill patients being admitted to hospital should be a routine part of medical assessment, an editorial in the journal declared.

HEALTH PROBLEMS DUE TO DRINK
Illnesses associated with continued alcohol abuse are generally related to the effect it has on the body. It is claimed that about one-third of heavy drinkers suffer from chronic inflammation of the stomach lining, which results in loss of appetite, under-nourishment and – if aspirin is swallowed – increases the risk of gastric bleeding. Alcohol can cause cancer of the mouth, throat and gullet if consumed in large amounts over a period of time. Two recent American studies suggest a possible link between heavy drinking and breast cancer, but much more research is needed before such a connection can be firmly established. Australian research has shown that alcohol can also cause brain shrinkage, which appears to be reversible if heavy drinking is stopped. Some symptoms associated with alcohol – notably headaches – are caused by artificial additives included to provide drinks with a characteristic taste, scent and colour (as in the case of red wine and port). Sexual and infertility problems affecting both men and women can also result from heavy drinking.

Nutritional deficiencies – especially those involving vitamins – are very common among heavy drinkers, who rely on alcohol to provide 'empty calories' but little else of dietary value. On the other hand, obesity – leading to an increased risk of high blood pressure and heart disease – can result from combining regular heavy drinking with normal eating habits. For example, the average person obtaining the standard quota of calories from food (2,000 per day for a woman, 2,500–3,000 for a man) may top up these amounts substantially through drink, especially if little physical exercise is taken. A pint of beer provides about 180 calories; a pint of light ale 150; a small whisky about 60; a glass of dry white wine 75; a glass of sweet white wine 100 calories.

DRINKING DURING PREGNANCY

Despite extensive research in Britain and other countries, doctors have found it impossible to say precisely that any small amount of alcohol can be regarded as safe for all expectant mothers. There is evidence that a large proportion of women now cut out drinking altogether during pregnancy and, where it is possible to plan ahead for a pregnancy, a great many now aim to stop drinking several months before conception. At the same time, doctors are anxious that mothers who drink moderately should not assume it is their fault if a baby is born below the average birth weight or is handicapped in some way, since these problems can be due to many other causes.

There is no doubt that, as in the case of other drugs taken by the mother, alcohol does pass through her bloodstream to the foetus in the womb. Research suggests that quite small amounts of alcohol taken regularly can affect the unborn baby's growth rate and birth weight, and can increase risk of miscarriage. The most serious complication of heavy drinking during pregnancy is, of course, 'foetal alcohol syndrome' (FAS), a relatively rare condition in which the baby suffers from very severe physical malformations and usually mental retardation. It has been shown that FAS occurs only in cases where the mother has been a chronic drinker with an intake of at least 80 grams of alcohol a day (about eight glasses of table wine or four large whiskies) before and during pregnancy. That is not to say that all heavy drinkers will automatically have babies affected by FAS. What it does mean is that expectant mothers who are worried should stop drinking, arrange to see their doctor immediately, and give an honest account of their alcohol intake, since they may need extra care throughout pregnancy.

DIAGNOSING ALCOHOL PROBLEMS

Ascertaining which patients have an alcohol problem is rarely an easy task for the GP or hospital doctor who first meets them when they seek advice for seemingly unrelated complaints. Even when asked a straightforward question, heavy drinkers are notoriously shy about admitting to a serious problem, even to themselves. So, with increasing experience, doctors are learning not to take replies mentioning 'an occasional drink' or 'a few drinks' at their face value, and are devising indirect methods of questioning which are likely to provide more accurate information, when they suspect that a problem may be related to heavy drinking.

Simple questionnaires designed to pick out acknowledged pointers to alcohol abuse are now frequently used for this purpose. Replies which highlight difficulties in several aspects of life can be very revealing, since people with serious drink problems are much more likely to have debts, difficulties in marriage and at work, to get into trouble because of aggressive behaviour and to find themselves accused of offences against the law. Physical indications include digestive troubles, neurological problems (such as numbness, tingling and shaking in the limbs) and a history of frequent accidental injuries. The latter finding has led to the development of a simple five-point 'trauma questionnaire' by researchers in Ontario, Canada, and Cleveland, Ohio, who report that over two-thirds of early alcohol abusers can be identified through its use combined with conventional blood tests. The questions are as follows:

'Since your 18th birthday: (1) Have you had any fractures or dislocations in your joints? (2) Have you been injured in a road traffic accident? (3) Have you injured your head? (4) Have you been injured in an assault or fight (excluding injuries during sport)? (5) Have you been injured after drinking?' The more 'yes' answers, the greater the probability of an alcohol problem.

One of the simplest and reputedly most successful screening devices for detecting 'hidden alcoholics' in the doctor's surgery is the CAGE questionnaire, which asks

four questions:
'(1) Have you ever felt that you ought to cut down on your drinking?
(2) Have people annoyed you by criticising your drinking?
(3) Have you ever felt bad or guilty about your drinking?
(4) Have you ever had a drink first thing in the morning, to steady your nerves or get rid of a hangover?'

The value of such questionnaires as a guide to self-help seems obvious. It is well known that the most difficult part of seeking and accepting help for problem drinking (and for other addictions) is the basic problem of admitting to oneself that help is needed. With a simple structured questionnaire like the CAGE, it is virtually impossible to be untruthful with yourself – if you have a drink problem. It is this moment of truth which is the turning point for the many who, through organizations like Alcoholics Anonymous, do find their way from addiction to recovery.

GETTING HELP
Most people who wish to cut back on drinking are moderate drinkers, who, once they understand the limits regarded as safe, are able to reduce their intake of their own accord. At the other extreme, those with serious problems involving regular or periodic heavy drinking may find that the only solution is to stop drinking altogether, with the support of Alcoholics Anonymous and, ideally, under medical supervision. Between these two levels of alcohol consumption are the large group of moderate to moderately heavy drinkers who feel a need to reduce their consumption without necessarily giving up drinking altogether, but are unsure how to proceed.

Let us assume that through social pressures or for some other reason you have gradually drifted into this middle category of drinkers. The first question to ask is, how would you know? One sign is that you have begun to feel guilty and furtive about your drinking, because you are spending more time and money on it than you consider reasonable. You find yourself repeatedly drinking more than you had intended and, at odd times, 'longing' for a drink in a way that worries you. Instead of seeing a drink as a pleasant accompaniment to a chat with friends at your local, now it is the main attraction of such get-togethers. If you can manage it, you try to sneak in an extra drink between rounds. You've got into the habit of drinking at home during the day. It takes more alcohol than formerly to give your spirits a 'lift', but less to make you feel inebriated. You are missing meals and feeling irritable, and your moods are interfering in your relationships with others. You are likely to answer 'yes' to two or three of the four key questions in the CAGE questionnaire described above.

Facing up to the fact that you have a drink problem is the first step in coming to grips with it. Once you have the will to reduce your intake, then you are ready to find the answers to some crucial questions which will help you to regain control:

- In what circumstances did I start drinking too much?
- Where do I do most drinking?
- At what time of day am I likely to drink most?
- Do I just want to cut down my drinking or is my problem so serious that I can manage only if I stop altogether?
- Do I think I need medical advice?
- Would it help to talk to a counsellor or someone in a self-help group about my problem?
- Take a written note of your questions and answers for future reference.

Most of us live our lives by a routine of some sort, and it is within this sort of time structure that we are likely to find the key to our own behaviour. Unless we are completely disorganized, we find that we 'fit in' recreational activities according to the time available. And because we all tend to be 'creatures of habit', it doesn't always occur to us to switch to some other activity once an old habit has lost is novelty or has begun to cause concern. A case in point is the pint at lunch time, and perhaps another 'jar' or two at the end of the day, which can extend into an evening's drinking if you are not careful. The answer is to find something else which is even more enjoyable than a chat in the pub at lunch-time, and to establish a different routine for the early evening which does not leave time for more than one drink in the pub near your workplace.

However difficult this solution may seem at first glance, it is one which works for a great many people who are worried enough about their drinking to want to 'change their lives'. For many younger people, the answer is physical exercise, and fortunately opportunities for this are available everywhere these days. Nick, a 32-year-old accountant, explains how he came to spend his lunch breaks on the squash court: 'I don't think I had much of a drink problem, but I really was very unfit – quite flabby and with the beginnings of a beer belly. One day I just happened to glance at the notices in the library near where I work and realized that there were squash courts nearby which were open at lunch time, and that is how it began. I was lucky in that two of the people I used to drink with were also interested, because it takes a bit more effort to make the change on your own.'

'Everyone knows that exercise is good for you, but I don't think they realize how beneficial it can be mentally as well as physically,' says Paula, a physical education teacher who runs an aerobics class for women in her spare time. 'Most of those I see are women who don't go out to work or are unemployed, and a great many of them start out with problems like overweight, depression, drinking too much, and you can see that they are very low in self-esteem. The big stumbling-block is getting them to come a second time, because if they do they will persevere. Once they've sorted themselves out physically and are able to keep up with the exercise programme, they begin to feel more in control of other aspects of their lives, and to get back their self-respect. This is very true of the women with drink problems.'

Relaxation is another powerful ally for anyone trying to bring a drinking problem under control or learning to cope with emotional difficulties of some kind. Information about classes can be obtained from local advice centres but, for someone trying to overcome a drink problem at home during the day, having a relaxation tape-recording on hand can be a big help when the temptation to have a drink has to be resisted.

For many women, the most valuable help is found

through membership of a self-help group, where success is achieved through mutual support and understanding. Women's health groups usually provide support for those with a wide variety of problems. All such groups find that there are immense therapeutic benefits to be gained through working together, and exploring the reasons for drinking or other self-damaging behaviour – smoking, illicit drug abuse, serious overeating problems, gambling or compulsive shoplifting.

One of the best sources of information on controlling drinking and on local help services is Alcohol Concern, a national charitable organisation. They also provide some tips to help you drink in safety:

- Think in units and, if necessary, keep a drink diary.
- Pace your drinks so that you drink no more than one unit an hour of alcohol, and alternate with soft drinks.
- Drink more slowly so that you drink less.
- Don't be afraid to say no to an offer of another drink.
- Don't drink on an empty stomach.
- Don't buy rounds – it's better to say you will buy your own drink.
- Have days off so that you have at least two or three alcohol-free days a week.
- At home don't exceed the standard pub measures when you pour a drink.
- Never drink and drive or accept a lift from a driver who has been drinking.
- If you're giving a party offer plenty of soft drinks and don't force alcohol on your guests – even at the risk of appearing mean.
- Avoid activities which can be dangerous if you have been drinking, such as operating machinery, swimming or sailing.

CHAPTER 8

Drug treatment for depression

At first glance, the doctor's task in prescribing for someone complaining of depression may seem a relatively simple one, yet there are a number of considerations to be taken into account. In a case of simple reactive depression, it may be decided that counselling or a short course of psychotherapy – if such help is available – would be preferable to medication.

It may not always be easy for the doctor at a first consultation to assess to what extent anxiety is a feature of the patient's depression, yet this distinction is important when it comes to selecting a drug which is likely to be most helpful. If, on the other hand, the patient seems lethargic and listless, a different type of drug may be more suitable.

Once depression has been diagnosed, knowing the nature of the depression itself can be a further aid to the prescribing doctor, and it usually helps if the patient can provide information about any previous episodes of a similar illness. However, since reactive, endogenous and manic depression tend to have similar symptoms in the early stages, the first choice of treatment is usually a tricyclic anti-depressant; if one drug in this group fails to provide relief after several weeks, another drug may be more successful.

The ideal anti-depressant would be one which provided rapid relief with the minimum of side-effects; but even with newer tricyclics and related drugs, it usually takes at least a week before any anti-depressant effect is felt and it may take considerably longer before full relief is experienced. As a rule, doctors and pharmacists warn patients that such delay is to be expected, as well as some initial side-effects which can safely be ignored. But depressed persons are not always able to concentrate fully on the advice they are given or to remember what has been said. Consequently, a great many stop their medication prematurely before it has had time to have a beneficial effect, or because of some mild side-effect which is not fully understood. Except where there is a serious reaction when medication should be stopped immediately, it is usually wiser to consult the doctor before stopping treatment.

Since drugs used to treat depression and anxiety may have an effect on your ability to concentrate and on muscle coordination, especially in the initial stages of treatment, you should ask your doctor for advice about the wisdom of driving a car or using delicate or dangerous equipment before starting such therapy. As your own GP is likely to be the only doctor who has full knowledge of your treatment, you should always inform any other doctor or dentist who is about to treat you of any drugs you are already taking, including herbal remedies, to avoid interaction with other drugs, including some anaesthetic substances. Obviously, this advice is especially important if you need treatment for any reason while away on holiday.

In the following lists, which are as complete as possible at the time of writing, drugs are identified by their British trade names. These are the names usually used on prescriptions and containers supplied by the chemist. In other countries, different trade names are sometimes used for these drugs so you should check with the prescribing doctor or pharmacist if you are worried about any apparent discrepancy.

DRUGS
Tricyclic anti-depressants
This group includes *sedatives* for depression with anxiety (Tryptizol, Domical, Lentizol, Prothiaden, Sinequan, Surmontil, Triptafen, Limbitrol); and non-sedatives for depression with lethargy (Elavil, Evadyne, Anafranil, Pertofran, Gamanil, Tofranil, Allegron, Aventyl, Prondol, Concordin).

Note
It usually takes from seven to ten days for these to produce

any noticeable effect, and from four to six weeks for compete relief. Common side-effects include dryness of the mouth, nausea, constipation, drowsiness, dizziness, increased sweating and reduced libido. Because they sometimes have an effect in lowering blood-pressure and causing changes in heart rhythm, regular medical checks are advisable. Since they can cause drowsiness, patients who drive a car may be advised to take these drugs before going to bed.

Other drugs with which these may react adversely include alcohol, amphetamines, appetite suppressants which act on the central nervous system, antihistamines (found in common cold treatments, anti-allergy preparations and travel sickness pills), MAOI anti-depressants (see pages 142-143), and some anaesthetics. Dentists and hospital doctors should be told before starting treatment if someone is taking these drugs. Tricyclics should not be given to pregnant women. Doctors are also advised to be cautious in prescribing them for anyone with disorders of the heart, liver or thyroid gland, for those suffering from diabetes, epilepsy and psychotic illness, and for lactating women.

To avoid withdrawal symptoms, tricyclics should be reduced gradually over several weeks when ending treatment. Withdrawal symptoms – which usually depend on dosage and length of use and tend to be more severe with longer-established versions of these drugs – can include anxiety, panic attacks, sleep disturbance with vivid dreams, restlessness, weakness, muscle pain and gastro-intestinal problems.

Second generation anti-depressants
These are newer drugs with similar action to tricyclics, but differing from them chemically and said to have fewer side-effects. They include: Ludiomil, Bolvidon, Norval, Molipaxin, Vivalan.

Tricyclic combinations
These drugs are intended for patients suffering from both anxiety and depression. One of those listed (Limbitrol) includes a minor tranquillizer. Three others (Motipress, Motival, Triptafen) incorporate major tranquillizers.

Note

The main side-effects of these drugs are similar to those for tricyclic anti-depressants. *Minor tranquillizers* (Librium, Valium, Stelazine, etc.) can in some cases intensify existing depression; they should be stopped gradually to avoid withdrawal symptoms. *Major tranquillizers* (stronger anti-psychotic drugs) can cause dryness of the mouth, muscle stiffness, trembling of the hands and more severe neurological symptoms if taken over a long period.

MAOI anti-depressants

The group of drugs known as MAOIs or 'monoamine oxidase inhibitors' are so called because they limit the body's ability to deal with certain natural substances called amines, which are normally involved in processing stress-related chemicals like adrenaline and noradrenaline. In this way they can be very effective in relieving depression and stress. They include Nardil, Marsilid, Marplan, Parnate and Parstelin. However, these drugs have the disadvantage that, in addition to the desired effect, they also block the action of other chemicals which the body normally uses to process certain food and drink constituents and other drugs, including tricyclic anti-depressants. If taken in combination with MAOIs, these can lead to dangerously high blood pressure and very severe headache – a symptom which should be reported to the doctor at once.

Because of this risk, a doctor prescribing MAOIs will supply a list of foods which must *not* be eaten because they contain the amine – tyramine – which the body can no longer process efficiently. Banned foods include meat and yeast extracts (Bovril, Marmite and other brands), cheese, yoghurt, chocolate, bananas, avocado, broad bean pods, some vegetable protein products and pickled foods. Drinks which must not be taken include beer and some wines, especially Chianti. Banned drugs include other anti-depressants, antihistamines, common cold cures, narcotic analgesics (such as pethidine), atropine, amphetamines and barbiturates. Fourteen days should be allowed to elapse after stopping an MAOI drug before taking any of the above-mentioned substances.

The warning card supplied by the prescribing doctor

should be carried at all times and be shown to any doctor or dentist who is about to provide treatment for any reason. MAOIs should be stopped gradually to avoid withdrawal symptoms, which can include headache, nausea, shivering, sweating, panic attacks and disturbing nightmares, especially if the drug has been taken for nine months or longer.

Having fallen from favour for some years because of the danger to patients involved in their ignoring instructions, MAOIs are again becoming more popular among doctors. Their advantage is that they can often provide relief from severe depression where other anti-depressants have failed. Some specialists remain sceptical, on the basis that safety depends too much on patients always remembering to comply with essential restrictions, especially as forgetfulness is often a characteristic of depression. They warn that in careless hands MAOIs are the most dangerous anti-depressants available, and the need for the strictest care in avoiding forbidden food and drinks does not always rest only with the patient, of course. Family and friends also need to be on the alert to ensure that a banned ingredient is never used in a dish to be shared by a person taking MAOI drugs. If banned foods or drink have been taken inadvertently, treatment should be stopped until the doctor has been consulted.

Other anti-depressants
These include Fluanxol, a low-dose version of an anti-psychotic drug which is given for anxiety and depression; caution is needed if used by anyone with severe heart, liver or kidney disease. Optimax and Pacitron are both given for manic-depression; they should not be combined with MAOI drugs or taken by anyone with bladder disease. Xanax, a member of the benzodiazepine group of minor tranquillizers, is given for anxiety and depression; it may cause dependence and should be withdrawn gradually.

Lithium salts anti-depressants
Camcolit, Liskonum, Litarex, Phasal, Priadel are usually prescribed for manic-depression. Lithium therapy has

proved very effective in the long-term prevention of
recurrent symptoms and may be used in combination with
tricyclic anti-depressants. Where other drugs have failed to
provide relief in endogenous depression lithium has also
proved effective, but because it is a potentially toxic
substance, which tends to lower the level of sodium salts in
the body and to alter the body's fluid balance, it can be used
only under close medical supervision. In practice, this
means that regular checks on the level of lithium in the
blood are an essential part of treatment. Usually, these start
one week after the treatment has begun. Other drugs
which interact with lithium include diuretics (to increase
urinary excretion), theophylline (for respiratory treatment)
and non-steroidal drugs (NSAIDS) for rheumatic conditions. The drug should not be given to anyone suffering
from kidney failure.

It is of particular importance to report without delay any
side-effects which may be associated with this treatment.
Mild side-effects can include tiredness, muscle tremor and
gastro-intestinal problems. Increased urinary excretion
may be another side-effect, underlining the necessity to
avoid drugs like diuretics and theophylline, which have
this effect. Severe adverse effects and toxic effects can
include drowsiness, vomiting, diarrhoea, and under-
activity of the thyroid gland (signs of the latter condition
can include loss of appetite and energy, lowered body
temperature, marked dryness of the skin and mental
dullness.) *Lithium should be stopped at once* and the doctor
should be consulted if any of these severe adverse effects is
experienced.

ECT SHOCK TREATMENT FOR DEPRESSION
ECT (electro-convulsive therapy) may be offered to
severely depressed patients who have not responded to
other forms of treatment, or who cannot tolerate the
side-effects of anti-depressant drugs. These may include
sufferers from endogenous and manic depression –
especially very elderly patients – and patients recognised as
having a high suicide risk who need treatment capable of
inducing a rapid change in mood. Another group

frequently offered ECT are severely depressed people with serious eating disorders, for whom a change of mood can also be a life-saver. Although the technique has been the centre of controversy for many years, many psychiatrists and patients testify to its value where other approaches have failed. 'For me, it was a life-saver. It brought instant relief when I was at my lowest ebb,' says 30-year-old Suzanne.

In its modern modified form, ECT is a very much refined version of the cruder operation pioneered in Italy some fifty years ago. Electrodes are attached to one or both temples, and a low-voltage electric current is passed through the brain for a fraction of a second. A short-acting intravenous anaesthetic is given beforehand, together with a muscle-relaxant drug to counteract convulsive movements produced by the shock. The patient regains consciousness within twenty minutes, and then sleeps for about an hour. A typical course of treatment, which may be combined with anti-depressant drugs, consists of between six and twelve sessions at a rate of two or three a week on a hospital out-patient basis. Sometimes women miss one or two periods while having a course of ECT. However, the most troublesome problem associated with the treatment is loss of memory of events and information acquired around the time of treatment. Specialists claim that recovery from this form of amnesia occurs rapidly, once the course is completed.

ECT is believed to work through an effect on the brain chemistry involved in depression predominantly due to biological causes. Immediate relief may follow a single treatment for endogenous or manic depression, and the method has been found successful in treating elderly patients with seasonal depression. A success rate as high as 70 to 80 per cent has been reported for ECT.

Not all patients are helped by ECT, however. Most sufferers from reactive depression are less likely to benefit; and indeed some distinguished psychiatrists have advocated using ECT as a diagnostic tool so that non-responders could be identified as suffering from reactive depression. 'Such an approach, employed on a wide scale, accounts for the large number of people who at some time or another have had ECT for no other reason than that their psychiatrist thought it would not do any harm and might even cast light on the situation,' says Professor Anthony Clare. 'Not surprisingly, such patients look upon ECT with little favour and many of them spend some time and effort denigrating ECT as a degrading and useless form of treatment.'

On the other hand, medical research and experience have made it possible to identify with considerable accuracy the type of patient who is most likely to benefit from ECT. A clinical profile predictive of a good response to ECT would include features such as a family history of depression, a history of weight loss, an illness of sudden onset with early morning wakefulness and of less than one year's duration, mental and physical 'retardation' (such as apathy), a sense of personal worthlessness, and a pyknic body build, tending to rotundity and fatness.

The term 'pyknic' was introduced early this century by the German psychiatrist, Ernst Kretschmer, to typify the body build most often associated with manic-depression. He considered that schizophrenia was more likely to occur in people of asthenic or narrow, slender body build, with a longer rib-cage than those of pyknic build. However, while these distinctions are of interest, they are not usually used as a diagnostic guide.

During the 1970s, ECT attracted a great deal of public criticism, largely on the grounds of over-use among long-stay hospital patients of a technique which seemed unacceptable at best and barbaric at worst. So is ECT safe? 'The risk of death with ECT is negligible,' according to Professor Clare. Standards in ECT practice are said to have improved in recent times, following a 1981 Royal College of Psychiatrists survey of 165 clinics, which found many shortcomings both in the equipment used and in clinic staffing. Clearly, past criticism was deserved in many cases.

DAYLIGHT TREATMENT
See phototherapy for seasonal affective disorder (pages 49-51).

SLEEP ADJUSTMENT THERAPY FOR DEPRESSION
Early morning wakefulness is a common characteristic of severe endogenous depression, and this is the time of day when the sufferer's mood tends to be at its most despairing. 'You wonder how you can ever make it to 10 a.m, as the most destructive thoughts crowd in to haunt you,' says Sheila, who is being treated for recurrent bouts of depression. 'You lie there reliving every bad moment in your life, every nasty remark anyone has ever made about you. But the worst part is remembering all the stupid things you've ever said or done – incidents probably long forgotten by the others involved.'

Biological or endogenous depression is understood to be due to some imbalance in the brain chemistry involved in mood regulation. An explanation for early waking is that it is related to disturbances in circadian rhythms, the body-clock mechanism which operates in a 24-hour or 25-hour cycle and involves most of the body's physiological activity. The idea of treating this problem by resetting the body-clock through temporary sleep-deprivation was first put to the test by a German researcher in 1971. He reported favourable results when a group of depressed patients was kept awake continuously for 36 hours, but in this and later studies improvement proved to be only of short duration. Since then, other approaches have been tried.

Sleep-deprivation is believed to have an anti-depressant effect by eliminating REM (rapid eye movement) dream periods. These can be detected in a sleep laboratory by encephalography (EEG brain-wave tracings). More recent American studies have involved waking the sleeper before REM sleep occurs, then readjusting sleep patterns to persuade the body-clock to extend its activity to a slightly longer day, with apparent success in terms of relief from early waking. However, this method has the drawback that it is difficult to use outside a sleep laboratory. Some experts question its usefulness, in any case, on the basis that other factors besides dreams (such as recent weight loss) are also related to REM sleep patterns. Moreover, tricyclic anti-depressants and in some cases MAOIs can have a powerful effect in suppressing REM sleep, so that relief of depression may sometimes be due to drugs rather than to sleep-deprivation. Nevertheless, Sheila finds that staying up until after midnight, no matter how tired she feels, does help to shorten her own experience of the 'dawn blues'.

CHAPTER 9

Talking treatment

In a psychoanalytic case history recorded a hundred years ago by Freud and his colleague Joseph Brever, their famous patient, Anna O, is credited with originating the term 'talking cure'.

It does seem to be true that most people are helped to some extent by talking treatment, and a great many people benefit considerably. Family doctors who are able to provide counselling or therapy, by having the services of a part-time counsellor, social worker or community psychiatric nurse, have reported favourably on their experiences. For one thing, patients receiving therapy tend to need fewer prescriptions for anti-depressants and tranquillizers. Another consideration is that to have 'someone to talk to', who has time to listen and the capacity to understand, is often a healing process in itself. Obviously a lot depends on the personalities of client and therapist, and whether they can establish a good working relationship. This is important in any kind of partnership, and may take time to achieve.

Professional help available through the National Health Service, through a voluntary organization or privately includes counselling and psychotherapy (see lists on pages 171-182). Counselling is the easier to obtain; psychotherapy, under the National Health Service, is a relatively scarce resource, so that patients referred for this treatment are usually those with more severe problems.

Both of these approaches involve conversations between client and therapist, in which experiences, thoughts, feelings and relationships are explored with a view to clarifying the client's understanding of his situation and to help him resolve any emotional conflicts which may be contributing to his problems. Both counsellors and psychotherapists who work in the NHS and for reputable organisations outside it must have completed a recognized course of training. Many already have qualifications in psychology, nursing or social work and, of course, many are also medically qualified. Many qualified counsellors and therapists work privately and, if you need to find one, your best approach is through the recommendation of another professional in the area or through one of the organizations listed on pages 171-182.

You may be lucky enough to live in an area where there are facilities for 'walk in' inquiries, self-referrals and free counselling and therapy services. Fees for private therapy can vary considerably. It is always worth while discussing the possibility of a lower fee when starting treatment, especially if this involves long-term therapy which is likely to continue for a year or longer.

One criticism of psychotherapy is that while it can help to alleviate distress and 'cure' emotional ills, it does nothing to change the social evils which so often are the main cause of breakdown and subsequent relapse. Perhaps this is taking too gloomy a view of life after therapy, in which it is assumed that the client must continue to exist in the same emotional vacuum as before. It does not have to be like that. This is the point at which many clients rediscover their strengths, feel the urge to help others through self-help groups or voluntary work, or find new directions for themselves in a change of career. In the process, they are doing their best to make the world a better place for themselves and for many others.

MUTUAL HELP GROUPS
Without realizing it, we all make use of 'talking treatment' of some kind. When in 1973 the National Association for Mental Health used this term as the title for one of its helpful pamphlets, the subject under discussion was counselling and psychotherapy, both forms of treatment involving a course of conversations with a specially qualified professional. We should also remember that talking treatment can work on an everyday basis and in the context of self-help groups.

Obviously, you don't have to be emotionally disturbed or to have insurmountable social problems to benefit from the sort of 'confiding relationship' which can be a major barrier against depressive illness. Everyone needs 'someone to talk to' from time to time, someone to trust, who is a good listener, slow to condemn, sparing with the sort of advice which suggests easy solutions to complex problems yet wise enough to provide a clearer perspective. These are the qualities people have always looked for when seeking the counsel of others more experienced than themselves.

The concept of self-help means not only learning from our own experience but having an open mind so that we can learn from the experience of others, and having the humility to recognize that we need this sort of external support. To a large extent, the modern self-help group has taken the place previously occupied by the 'extended family' of parents, grandparents and other near relatives living close at hand, through which former generations of young people acquired their 'coping skills'.

Today, in most areas, you are likely to find mutual support groups catering not only for those with specific problems but also for those at risk through the effects of loneliness and isolation. These can include young mothers living in high-rise blocks, working girls in cheerless bed-sits, bachelors with no source of companionship except the pub, old people living alone, divorced and bereaved people, and so on.

For many of those with mental health problems, a self-help group often provides the only opportunity they have to discuss their problems in depth with another person and to discover that they are not alone in their distress. It is essential to remember that membership of a group is not all one-sided: while each member gains support from the others, in turn each member also *gives* support, so that the 'pool' of insight and wisdom available through a good group can be considerable. Another advantage is the loyalty and commitment which many groups inspire, so that long-standing members often remain to guide and contribute long after their own personal problems have been resolved.

151

This is very true of recovery and personal growth movement fellowships which have adapted the philosophy and spiritual orientation of Alcoholics Anonymous for their own programmes. The best known are Al-Anon for families of problem drinkers and Narcotics Anonymous and Families Anonymous for illicit drug users and their relatives, and others run along similar lines. There is no doubt that much of the success of these groups stems from the expertise which members acquire in interpreting the individual guidelines for each group and in helping newcomers to help themselves, by encouraging them to develop a more positive outlook on life and to see their problems in a different perspective. As an Al-Anon member puts it: 'We may not be able to change your problem, but we can help you to change the way in which you think about it so that you are better able to cope with it.'

One of the major advantages of groups inspired by the AA philosophy is that they provide a firm structure for the guidance of meetings, thus avoiding the risk of the group becoming little more than a social gathering. At the same time, their approach has a great deal in common with cognitive therapy in that it aims to change for the better the way in which members think about their problems.

An international community mental health movement incorporating these principles is GROW, which is relatively new to Britain but has a large membership in the United States, Australia, New Zealand, Ireland and other European countries. GROW was founded in Australia 30 years ago by Father Cornelius Keogh, a Jesuit priest who attended AA meetings after he had suffered a nervous breakdown. Convinced of the need for a similar non-denominational 'personal growth' movement geared to the needs of people with mental health problems, he decided to adopt some of AA's principles for a new mutual-help fellowship. In Britain, one of the longest-established groups is held in the Priory Hospital in London.

GROW is currently of particular interest because it is one of the very few mutual help or self-help groups to have its methods and achievements subjected to scientific study. A major research programme to investigate the effectiveness of GROW groups in America is being carried out by psychologists at the University of Illinois under the leadership of Professors Julian Rappaport and Edward Seidman, and their early findings have been highly favourable.

The team's first report showed that those who had been members of GROW for nine months or more were 'significantly better off' than members of only three months' standing, in terms of social adjustment, employment and mental health. In a report in *Social Policy* (Winter 1985), they summed up their impression of GROW's routine: 'Groups of between three and 15 members meet weekly for about two hours, and follow a structured "group method". Important components of the group method include personal testimonies, discussion of members' problems and progress, discussion of readings from the GROW literature, and assigning "practical tasks" and out-of-group contact between members for the coming week. Each group has an elected volunteer "organiser", whose role is to keep the group on task and consistent with GROW's principles. Each week the organiser selects a participant "leader" to run the meeting . . . The leaders are also the members. People are encouraged to take increasing responsibility as they become a part of the organisation.'

Most good self-help groups have an element of therapy and co-counselling, which means that as members gain insight they are able to help each other to see their problems in a clearer perspective and to find ways of coping with them. The basic principles of counselling can be learnt under the guidance of an experienced leader, a professional therapist, a community psychiatric nurse or a specialist social worker. Many groups, and especially those which are part of a national organization, have developed their own techniques for helping with specific problems which are usually broadly in line with professional practice.

Unless the group you are thinking of joining has an established reputation, it is advisable first to consult your doctor, social services department or nearest MIND branch. Ask your doctor's receptionist if there is a part-time counsellor or social worker attached to the practice and whether an appointment with either of these can be arranged. (You may not always find information about their availability posted up in the GP's waiting-room.) On the other hand, your doctor may already be working closely with a voluntary group which can be recommended.

No matter how impeccable the credentials of an organization, local branches may occasionally fall short of the newcomer's expectations. This is not surprising, since so much depends on the personalities of those involved, especially in leadership roles. It is important that you should feel 'at home' in the group from the start, and that you give yourself time to get to know the other members. Fortunately, experienced members soon realize when a meeting is getting off-course and can usually help to steer it in the right direction.

The sort of group best avoided is one where you find yourself being frightened off by too much bias in one direction or another. Dogmatic assertions such as, 'We have no time for doctors' or 'We are totally opposed to drugs of any kind' may well fit in with your own way of thinking, but they are designed to deter you from seeking out options which could be of benefit. Another warning signal is finding that other members are too eager to advise and make your decisions for you; this suggests that the basic principles of non-directive counselling are ignored or misunderstood.

Since virtually anyone is free to form a group or indeed set up as a therapist, it is possible to pick one which is promoting 'way-out' theories likely to add to your anxiety and confusion rather than relieve them. You cannot always accept at face value a group which seems to claim too much expertise, unless you know that the leader of the group is professionally trained. In one group I visited, the leader based his guidance completely on interpretation – or misinterpretation – of the psychoanalytic theories of Freud. Much to the exasperation of new members who wanted to talk about difficulties in relationships at work and such problems as phobic anxieties, he insisted on focusing on childhood conflicts and later sexual experiences. One man who, like me, had found the group through a newspaper advertisement, complained: 'I came here with what seemed to be a clear-cut problem of depression. Now I'm feeling more depressed than ever, because you've almost convinced me that I have some sort of personality conflict dating back to infancy. But I know *why* I'm depressed – it's because my girlfriend walked out on me.'

After the meeting I talked to a psychologist who was there as an observer. She explained that the group leader had no formal qualifications but had become interested in psychoanalysis when he was treated for a breakdown in the United States. 'He has read very widely on the subject, but he has no practical experience apart from his own illness and therapy, which is not a good starting point for trying to help others. Most of what goes on at these meetings seems to be fairly harmless because most of the members are "old hands" and tend to treat the proceedings as a sort of game or debating forum. The aspect I'm least happy about is where new people come along looking for help and perhaps reassurance, which they are unlikely to find here. A medical colleague and I are trying to get the leader to modify his approach on the grounds that it could be harmful for some people, and I think we are making some headway. Psychoanalytic theory is not something which unqualified people should be allowed to play around with. Anyway, psychoanalysis isn't always the most helpful type of treatment.'

There is no law to prevent anyone from starting a self-help or therapy group, especially where no charge is being made for services. 'The trouble is that some people who feel the urge to form a group are on an ego-trip of some kind or have problems of their own which haven't been completely resolved. In the average mutual help group, people with similar problems come together to share their experiences, but there is much less control where one individual with no training assumes a role of authority. Another risk for people who are already lonely and vulnerable is that they might be persuaded to join some obscure religious cult under the impression that they are going to receive realistic help with emotional and personal problems. My advice would be that no matter how

155

well-intentioned such people are or seem to be – 'and especially where money is likely to be involved – nobody should join up without having the group checked out with some responsible person in the neighbourhood or wider community.'

Apart from the professional sources of information listed on pages 171-182, local church leaders are in a key position to know what help is available locally and what is to be trusted. Indeed, most of the main churches in Britain are involved in providing welfare and counselling services on a non-denominational basis.

SETTING UP A SELF-HELP GROUP

It could happen, of course, that there is no group in your area which seems to meet your needs, but do not despair. This is the point at which you could begin to think seriously about helping to set up a new group, either for a specific purpose or one catering for people with a range of problems. For example, if you are interested in forming a group for sufferers from depression, phobias or anorexia, or relatives of problem drinkers, the best way to start is to contact the relevant national organization (see pages 173-176), or, if a more broadly-based group seems more suitable, then you might like to form a GROW branch (see page 175).

Clearly the prospect of taking such a step on your own is daunting, especially if you or some member of your family have an emotional problem of some kind. The answer is that you are unlikely to be on your own for very long, once you take the first step and begin to look around for prospective members. Unless you are able to work under the guidance of a national organization like MIND, the best places to look for help are the health services and social services departments (social *work* departments in Scotland). The social services department, in particular, is intimately concerned with community initiatives of all kinds since it has such a wide span of responsibilities – for children and young people, disabled and elderly people, mental health and mentally handicapped people, juvenile offenders and families with social problems.

The chances are that you know very little about the work

of your local authority's social services department, and would not know whom to contact. Telephone your town hall and ask to speak to someone in the information department who will be able to tell you if there is an individual or group within the service with whom you could discuss your proposed project. This might be someone with the title of community worker or mental health services co-ordinator, or someone with responsibility for a neighbourhood centre. Professionals such as these rely to a considerable extent on support from voluntary groups and may be able to help with accommodation for meetings. If you are lucky, the department may also be able to help with funds for your project.

A good way to learn about running a self-help group is to ask if you can sit in at meetings of other groups in your neighbourhood for single parenthood, unemployment, poor housing or some other social cause. You are bound to find one or two in which you can take a special interest. Liaising with other groups and getting to know all you can about local and national organizations can be a big help for your members once your own group has been launched. Finally, to preserve anonymity and privacy, it is best if only first names are used at meetings, and in letters to the local press, advertisements and notices in public libraries and other public premises to publicize your group and raise funds for stationery, postage, the use of a telephone and a share of the lighting bill for a shared premises.

COUNSELLING

Counsellors who work as therapists usually have qualifications recognized by the British Association for Counselling; others, whose expertise is in dealing with a specific problem, receive a more specialized form of training. At its best, counselling can often be as helpful as psychotherapy. An obvious test of the professional counsellor is that he or she very rarely offers advice. The counsellor's role is that of trusted listener and guide, who helps the client towards a clearer perspective on his problems and on the likely consequences of different courses of action which might be employed to deal with them, so that he is in a better position to make his own decisions.

Bereavement counselling is an example of counselling as therapy. This highly skilled approach is sometimes called for when a bereaved person is unable to come to terms with the loss of a loved one, and becomes severely depressed and anxious as a result. This is more likely to happen where grief is suppressed when someone dies, and, instead of 'working through' a normal period of mourning, the bereaved person bottles up his grief and may be unable to talk to anyone about his loss. Counselling can provide this desperately needed opportunity, so that the sufferer is able to live through grief and regain serenity of mind.

This type of counselling may involve up to six or more weekly sessions, each lasting about an hour. Family doctors can refer patients for free counselling under the NHS to a social worker or community psychiatric nurse with training in counselling, or to a hospital therapist, or there may be a suitable mutual help group in the area (see pages 173-176). Social workers are also involved in many counselling projects for which a medical referral is not needed and help is available on a voluntary basis.

PSYCHOANALYTIC PSYCHOTHERAPY

Psychoanalysis, the classic Freudian therapy which aims to promote healing through self-knowledge, provides the inspiration for psychoanalytic psychotherapy. Analysis works on the theory that neurotic illness is caused by conflict and maladjustment within the sufferer's own mind, and that these problems are traceable back to very early life experiences which the conscious mind has forgotten or cannot bear to remember. This type of treatment can be helpful for people with incapacitating neuroses who have serious difficulties with regard to relationships. It works less well for those with psychotic illnesses in which disorders of thought are a periodic feature.

One disadvantage of psychoanalysis is that it is not often available under the National Health Service. It is costly and time-consuming; it requires the services of a highly qualified therapist for as long as three years or even longer. Another criticism is that, while prolonged analysis can provide insight which is of benefit to the client, it may in some cases encourage an introspective attitude in which the client becomes excessively preoccupied with himself and his own reactions. During psychoanalytic psychotherapy, which is a modification of psychoanalysis, the client and therapist sit opposite each other (as opposed to having the patient reclining on the traditional couch) and can extend their discussions to include specific everyday life problems as well as deep-seated psychological difficulties. Unlike behavioural therapy, which works on the theory that behaviour is a learned response which can be 'un-learned', psychoanalytic psychotherapy sees self-destructive behaviour as originating in repressed thoughts hidden in the unconscious mind. In some cases, this therapy can be comparable to a full-scale analysis, depending on the client's needs. On average, however, it usually involves fewer sessions over a shorter period of time.

In an interview with medical writer Lindsay Knight, one therapist sums up the analytical approach: 'We look at people's difficulties in terms of their whole lives. It's not just a snapshot view of the present. Why, for instance, is this person prone to respond to adversity by always seeing themselves as unlovable or powerless? It is about finding some kind of hidden truth about how things are for you as an individual.' And a client gives her impression of her own therapist: 'I think she saved my life. It was amazing at first, at last there was someone who was there for me all the time. I could ring her if I was feeling really terrible and she saved me from two suicide attempts. She was someone who believed in me . . . I think everyone should have someone like her.' In a few words, these thumb-nail sketches tell us quite a lot about the value of psychotherapy for someone suffering from an illness such as severe depression.

While Freud's teaching is central to the principles of psychoanalytic psychotherapy, some of his theories have been modified by the distinguished workers in this field who came after him. This means in practice that therapists trained in different 'schools' may vary to some extent in their approach. For instance, an influential group sometimes described collectively as 'Neo-Freudians' considered that more emphasis should be placed on relationships and environmental influences in explaining neurotic illness. Jung tended to see neurosis as an attempt at self-treatment aimed at healing existing rifts in the mind and attaining a state of mystical calmness. Jung's analytic psychology has attracted a considerable following among 'seekers after wisdom' as well as people with emotional problems, but critics say it is too detached from everyday reality to benefit everyone who needs help. One of the most recent developments is feminist therapy, based mainly on psychoanalytic therapy while concentrating on the special needs of women, stemming from adverse social conditioning from an early age.

GROUP THERAPY
As distinct from work in the average self-help or mutual help group, group therapy involves the guidance of a therapist as leader, a method widely used in hospitals and other centres run by the National Health Service, where the main approach is based on analytic psychotherapy principles. Although this clearly is a much cheaper method than individual psychotherapy, there are other advantages to be gained through working in an effective group in which members provide therapy for each other. For those who have difficulty with relationships, the group promotes self-confidence in relating to others over a period, in a way that would not be possible in a one-to-one therapy relationship.

Psychodrama is an innovative technique used in many therapy groups, especially where difficulties in relationships with others feature prominently in clients' problems. Through unscripted role-playing, participants are able to act out situations which are a source of conflict for them personally under the guidance of a therapist, and with other members of the group playing the part of an influential person in this conflict. By acting out a conflict, the client is helped to understand the issues involved and learn better ways of dealing with them.

Transactional analysis is a form of group therapy carried out under the guidance of a qualified leader which focuses on the effect of the everyday 'transactions' which take place between people in the family circle, at work and in social relationships. TA's creator, Dr Eric Berne, was a Freudian psychoanalyst who saw the need to 'demystify' psychology so that its benefits could be extended more widely, and evolved this therapy to that end. In learning the language and principles of TA, group members also learn how early childhood experiences and impressions affect the way in which they currently relate to others, and how their response in 'inter-personal transactions' can be changed for the better. Some therapists work with NHS groups, but most work privately.

Family therapy is regarded as one of the best ways of helping to break down barriers to communication and improve understanding, when a member of the family suffers from a neurotic illness which is associated with disturbed relationships within the group. Family therapy is available on medical referral under the NHS. Clients for whom it is recommended may include children and adolescents who need help for emotional problems, and young people receiving treatment for problems such as solvent and drug abuse. This approach is a flexible one which allows one or sometimes two therapists to work with family members both on an individual and group basis, using a variety of therapy techniques.

Assertiveness training and social skills training are essentially behavioural therapy methods used by a therapist to help people with problems of poor self-confidence in dealing with relationships, or in facing up to difficult situations involving problems such as phobias. In this approach, therapy can involve role-playing designed to explore the reactions of group members in different circumstances, and 'modelling' in which the therapist demonstrates the most positive way for the client to react using re-learned behaviour. Where people with mental health problems could benefit from assertiveness training, this is likely to be available as part of a therapy programme. The technique is also being recognized increasingly as a valuable help for others who may be experiencing difficulties in personal and working relationships through lack of self-confidence. On this basis, assertiveness training classes are available through many schools and polytechnics, and through private tutors with special training.

Humanistic therapy is an 'umbrella' classification which includes many of the newer and 'alternative' therapies which became popular in the United States and Britain in the 1960s: primal therapy, Gestalt therapy, Rogerian therapy, transcendental meditation, and approaches developed by the human growth movement among them. Humanistic therapy places more emphasis on the spiritual aspects of human nature, and on the value of 'real self' fulfilment as a healing process. A great many people have been helped by these therapies, and many conventional psychotherapists tend to incorporate some of their techniques in their own work. It is not considered advisable, however, for people with mental health problems to join such groups without seeking the advice of their own doctor or therapist. This applies particularly to 'encounter groups' which tend to cater mainly for mentally healthy people who feel the need to seek more meaning in their lives.

BEHAVIOUR THERAPY

Whereas psychoanalytic psychotherapy looks for the causes of emotional problems in the unconscious mind and early experience, behaviour therapy adopts the more practical approach of looking at symptoms of disturbance which can be observed and are more accessible to treatment. Based on the educational theory that all behaviour is learned, the therapist helps the client to 'un-learn' disabling habits which have been acquired as part of a neurotic illness (see pages 56-100).

Behaviour therapy has the advantage that treatment can often be completed in a matter of months by concentrating on specific problems. While it does not usually attempt to probe for underlying emotional conflicts in anything like the same depth as psychoanalytic therapy, many behaviour therapists use some of the latter's techniques in helping clients to understand their illness. Behaviour therapy can work only if the client is motivated to cooperate fully with the therapist in working towards agreed goals on the road to recovery, and in carrying out carefully planned 'homework'.

More than most other therapies, behaviour therapy tends to be 'directive' in so far as the therapist adopts a teaching role. One of the basic techniques used in bringing behaviour under control is the teaching of relaxation, using breathing exercises, to induce a state of calmness. In some forms of behaviour therapy, hypnosis or hypnotherapy may be used as a more potent means of suggesting beneficial changes in behaviour – in cases where a compulsive urge is causing serious disruption of the client's life, for instance. Problems which can be helped by behaviour therapy include stammering, excessive shyness, anxiety, depression, and functional sexual problems (such as premature ejaculation in men and vaginal spasm in women) . It follows, therefore, that a great many patients referred for therapy under the NHS are being helped through behavioural techniques.

COGNITIVE BEHAVIOUR THERAPY
As the word 'cognitive' suggests, this form of therapy relates to what we know or *think* we know about ourselves and how we interpret events affecting our personal lives. Its aim is to help change negative and self-destructive thinking and attitudes where these are a feature of psychological problems, as often happens in depressive illness. The typical sufferer from severe depression tends to develop a negative attitude towards life, in which he sees himself as unloved and unlovable, focuses his attention on the negative aspects of everyday events, and regards adversities as a personal rebuff which he feels he deserves.

In cognitive therapy, the therapist helps the client to test each one of his damaging 'cognitions' in turn, so that he can judge for himself whether or not these have a basis in reality. Techniques which may be involved include 'thought catching' (in which clients are trained to monitor

and record their automatic thoughts) and encouraging
them to look for alternative interpretations of events for
which they believed they were to blame. A course of
treatment usually lasts from 12 to 20 weeks, where patients
are referred for hospital therapy. With the development of
primary health care in the community, and the attachment
of other professionals to general practices on a part-time
basis, many family doctors can now refer patients for
therapy, and there is evidence of increasing medical
interest in cognitive therapy, following on the pioneering
work of Dr Aaron Beck and Dr David Burns.

CHAPTER 10

Help yourself to think positively

The causes of emotional problems rarely are 'all in the mind', but it is in the mind that anguish is felt when things go wrong. And it is the mind which feeds and perpetuates the negative thinking patterns which are the hallmark of neurotic disorders. Thoughts are the implements through which anxiety, depression and morbid fears take hold and sap our initiative once we have allowed negative thinking a free rein. Yet it doesn't always have to be like this. We don't need to lose control, or allow destructive ideas to run riot and darken our days, as the experts quoted in this book have shown. Even if we have temporarily lost the habit of thinking positively, we can help ourselves towards a more constructive approach to life in general. Here are some suggestions for starting the process:

- Learn to relax more in everyday situations. Don't feel you have to worry about your problems and responsibilities all the time. Daydreaming helps to reduce anxiety and relaxes you mentally and physically. So do art, music, poetry, the company of animals, the scent of garden flowers. Don't think it is a waste of time to sit at ease or stand and stare; give your mind a much-needed holiday.

- Learn how to change your 'internal environment' and allow yourself 'space', when you feel tensed up and over-anxious. Rest with your muscles relaxed, close your eyes, and think of a pleasant scene you have known or glimpsed through a favourite poem or painting.

- Get out and about as much as you can, especially if you are feeling depressed. Even meandering around the local shops will do something to take your mind off your own troubles. Take a brisk walk every day. Get on your bike. Take up swimming, tennis or badminton. Exercise tones up mental as well as physical function.

- Identify the risk factors which trigger a bout of depression for you personally, and make a point of avoiding them. If you are desolate because of a recent parting, don't go on playing his favourite tune, wearing the perfume he liked, visiting scenes laden with sad memories. Dry your tears, turn your face to the future and learn to live again. Be firm in discouraging friends with a penchant for nostalgia who keep reminding you of the past. Persuade them instead to join you in fresh ventures, in breaking away from the old routine and in making new friends.

- When negative thoughts intrude, don't just sit there and allow them to take possession of your mind. Do something different at once to distract your attention. Switch on the radio, television set or a long-playing record. Practise aerobic exercises to music. Take the dog for a run (pets often are the best therapists, according to research). Mow the lawn. Do a spot of spring-cleaning.

- Follow the GROW group's 'Guidelines for objective thinking': I will go by what I know, not by how I feel. I will deal with behaviour, not motives, and interpret what others do and say in a calm and matter-of-course way, instead of dramatizing situations and attributing motives to them. I will keep a clear and steady view of what is important and what is unimportant in the events of life and personal relationships. I will avoid isolation and keep in friendly contact with other minds.

- If despondent thoughts keep you awake at night or early in the morning, don't lie there feeling hopeless, as is customary at such times. And don't worry about not sleeping. Keep a diverting novel or whodunnit on your bedside table. Make yourself a hot drink. Take a leisurely bath. Rest – if necessary on the living room couch – and use a suitable cassette tape to help you with relaxation exercises. If you still can't sleep, play some music, read some poetry or switch on to an early morning news programme.

- Learn a language or a new skill. There is something immensely satisfying about doing something to please yourself, especially if it promises to open up new horizons later. Brush up your rusty school French or Spanish or start on something completely new, through evening classes, tutorial records, and by tuning in to continental radio networks. You may never know unless you try that you have a hidden talent for music, painting or a craft or that you have a way with words as a writer or public speaker.

- Give yourself a laugh a day from reading, listening, talking or viewing. Laughter is the best medicine, the old adage tells us, and research has shown that humour does have a therapeutic effect on mind and body, presumably through stimulating production of endorphins, the body's own 'high'-inducing hormones.

- Have an occasional 'good cry' if you feel like it. Tears are one of nature's ways of releasing bottled-up emotional tensions. They are not a sign of weakness.

- Put more colour into your life. Colour psychology may be a new concept, but the idea that colours affect our mood is as old as the hills. It is thought to be due to impressions reaching the eye having an effect on brain chemistry. Studies have shown that yellow is the most cheering colour, red and orange the most stimulating, blues and greens the most relaxing, pink best for cooling anger, dark brown, deep purple and black the most depressing. If you can't change your entire decor, you can hang up some bright pictures at eye level (some larger public libraries have reproductions available on loan). Colour in the clothes you wear can both affect and reflect your mood, as it can in make-up, but here it's obviously a question of experimenting until you find what suits you, or of finding a store which offers special expertise in colour selection.

- Try to build up your self-esteem; in terms of emotional

well-being, your opinion of yourself is the only opinion
that really matters. Don't go on thinking that you are less
lovable, less competent, less worthwhile as a person just
because you feel rejected through the loss of a job or a
deserting spouse. Most people have these reactions in
similar situations. Console yourself that some losses
turn out to be blessings in disguise, leaving the way open
for opportunities you might otherwise have missed.

- Learn to be more self-assertive and self-confident. These
are qualities which can be taught and learned through
evening classes, women's mutual help and therapy
groups. Self-assertiveness training shows you how to
overcome shyness, hold your own in business and
personal relationships, express your feelings in a socially
acceptable form instead of bottling up anger and
frustration, and gain control over your life.

- Allow yourself a daily dose of success. Give yourself an
opportunity to develop your talents, aptitudes and
accomplishments. Join a society, evening class or other
venture which caters for a subject in which you can excel.
Paradoxically, being temporarily unemployed or prematurely retired can provide opportunities for self-
discovery for those who are able to shake off the
depression associated with these demoralizing conditions, and accept a new challenge.

- Take more interest in your community by joining a
cultural group, debating society or political party, and
insist on having your say. Participation helps to build up
your self-confidence; taking a back seat only increases
shyness and feelings of inadequacy. Check the notices in
your public library for information about local social
activities and opportunities for voluntary social work.
Involvements such as these are not only satisfying in
themselves, they also give you the chance to make new
friends and to develop new interests and a more positive
outlook.

Appendices

PROFESSIONAL HELPERS IN MENTAL HEALTH

GPs deal successfully with the majority of patients with mental health problems. A GP's referral is necessary for consultation with a psychiatrist, psychologist or psychotherapist under the National Health Service. Many GPs can refer patients to a counsellor or therapist who is attached to their own practice.

Psychiatrists are qualified doctors who have completed an additional course of specialist training in psychological medicine. Special skills which many use in treatment include psychoanalytic psychotherapy, hypnosis and behavioural therapy.

Psychogeriatricians are psychiatrists who specialize in mental health and mental disorder in elderly people.

Neurologists are specialists in disorders of the body's nervous system, which includes the brain and spinal cord, and the nerves' responsibility for various types of activity throughout the body. Examples of neurological disorders are multiple sclerosis, Parkinson's disease and dementia. Some neurological disorders, such as dementia, can give rise to symptoms of mental disorder through disturbance of brain function.

Psychologists are not usually medically qualified, although many have the title of 'Doctor' acquired through a PhD degree awarded on completion of advanced studies. Their special expertise is in the study of the mind in health and illness and in understanding human behaviour. Clinical psychologists, who have completed an additional training, usually work in NHS hospitals and clinics where they may be involved in assessment and diagnosis and in decisions

169

relating to treatment. Many psychologists based in hospitals, the community (usually attached to social services departments) and in private practice provide psychoanalytic and behavioural psychotherapy. Many others work in education, industry and other fields.

Psychiatric nurses have completed a course of specialist training, and are usually based in hospitals and clinics where they are involved in patient care, medical treatment and therapy programmes. Many nurses take additional training to qualify as nurse therapists, especially in behavioural psychotherapy. Some nurse therapists work in the community, usually with general practitioners. *Community psychiatric nurses* are psychiatric nurses who have completed additional training to prepare them for work in the community. Some CPNs are attached to psychiatric hospitals and psychiatric units in general hospitals, and their main responsibility is to provide support for former patients living in the community. Others work closely with GPs, who can refer patients to them for counselling and psychotherapy.

Social workers are professionals who have completed a recognized training leading to the Certificate of Qualification in Social Work. Many work in hospitals; others work in the education welfare service and for voluntary agencies. The majority work for the local authority social services department (social work department in Scotland), where they have a wide range of responsibilities for clients including those with mental health problems and their families. Some social workers provide counselling and psychotherapy in the community, often working closely with GPs. Others who are designated 'Approved Social Workers' under the 1983 Mental Health (Amendment) Act (Mental Health Officers in Scotland) have statutory duties and powers in relation to mentally ill people for whom compulsory hospitalization is being sought by doctors and relatives.

Occupational therapists are trained professionals with special skills in the use of activity to promote physical and mental well-being, and to rehabilitate patients suffering from physical and mental illnesses in preparation for life in the community. Many work in general hospitals with patients recovering from accidental injuries and disabling illnesses such as stroke. A large number work in psychiatric hospitals and clinics, and some others are employed in the community by social services departments. For mentally ill people, the scope of occupational therapy has been extended very substantially in recent years, as the role of creative activity in improving self-confidence and expanding intellectual horizons has become more widely recognized.

In an ideal situation, patients should be able to choose from a wide range of activities, such as art and drama therapy, music, movement and dance therapy, horticulture therapy, indoor and outdoor sports, discussion groups and exercise programmes. Experience and research have shown the value of all of these in restoring mental well-being, where occupational therapists or specialist teachers can provide such facilities. The sad reality is, however, that owing to the chronic shortage of resources in all mental health services, relatively few patients have all these choices open to them.

NATIONAL INFORMATION AND SUPPORT SERVICES
Age Concern England, 60 Pitcairn Road, Mitcham, Surrey CR4 3LL. Tel. (01) 640 5431.
Age Concern Northern Ireland, 128 Great Victoria Street, Belfast BT2 7BG. Tel. (0232) 245729.
Age Concern Scotland, 33 Castle Street, Edinburgh EH2 3DW. Tel (031) 225 5000.
Age Concern Wales, 1 Park Grove, Cardiff CF1 3BJ. Tel. (0222) 371566.
Association of Carers, First Floor, 21-23 New Road, Chatham, Kent ME4 4QS.
Association of Community Health Councils, 254 Seven Sisters Road, London N4 2HZ. Tel. (01) 272 5459.
British Epilepsy Association, Crowthorne House, Bigshotte, New Wokingham Road, Wokingham, Berkshire RG11 3AY. Tel. (0344) 773122.
College of Health, 18 Victoria Park Square, London E2 9PF.

Tel. (01) 980 6263. Has register of over 1,000 organizations from which information is available to college members. The college's Healthline – Tel. (01) 980 4848 – is free to everyone, and includes over 150 audio tapes on physical and mental health.

Gingerbread, 35 Wellington Street, London WC2E 7BN. Tel. (01) 240 0953. For one-parent families.

Help the Aged, St James Walk, London EC1. Tel. (01) 253 0253.

Mastectomy Association of Great Britain, 26 Harrison Street, London WC1H 8JG. Tel. (01) 837 0908.

Medical Advisory Service, 10 Barley Mow Passage, London W4 4PH. Tel. (01) 994 9874. A new charitable organization offering a 24-hour telephone service.

Mental After-Care Association, 110 Jermyn Street, London SW1Y 6HB. Tel. (01) 839 5953.

Mental Health Association of Ireland, 2 Herbert Avenue, Dublin 4. Tel. Dublin 695375.

Mental Health Foundation, 8 Hallam Street, London W1N 6DH. Tel. (01) 580 0145/6.

MIND (National Association for Mental Health), 22 Harley Street, London W1N 2ED. Tel. (01) 637 0741.

NACRO (National Association for Care and Rehabilitation of Offenders), 169 Clapham Road, London SW9 OPU. Tel. (01) 582 6500.

National Association of Citizens Advice Bureaux, 115 Pentonville Road, London N1. Tel. (01) 833 2181.

National Council for Carers and their Elderly Dependants, 29 Chilworth Mews, London W2 3RG. Tel. (01) 724 7776.

National Council for One-Parent Families, 255 Kentish Town Road, London NW5 2LX. Tel. (01) 267 1361.

National Council for Voluntary Organizations, 26 Bedford Square, London WC1B 3HU. Tel. (01) 636 4066.

National Federation of Self-Help Organizations, 150 Townmead Road, Fulham, London SW6 2RA. Tel. (01) 731 4438.

National Schizophrenia Fellowship, 78 Victoria Road, Surbiton, Surrey KT6 4NS. Tel. (01) 390 3651/2/3.

National Schizophrenia Fellowship (Northern Ireland), Room 6, Bryson House, Bedford Street, Belfast BT2 7FE.

Tel. (0232) 248006.

National Schizophrenia Fellowship (Scotland), 40 Shandwick Place, Edinburgh EH2 4RT. Tel. (031) 226 2025.

Northern Ireland Association for Mental Health, 84 University Street, Belfast B17 3JR. Tel. (0232) 228474.

Patients Association, Room 33, 18 Charing Cross Road, London WC2H 0HR. Tel. (01) 240 0671.

Psychiatric Rehabilitation Association, 21a Kingsland High Street, London E8 2JS. Tel. (01) 254 9753.

Rape Crisis Centre, PO Box 69, London WC1. Tel. (01) 837 1600 (24-hour service); (01) 278 3956 (office). See telephone directory for local services.

Samaritans, Central London 24-hour service: Tel. (01) 283 3400. Office hours only: (01) 938 1051. See local telephone directory for 24-hour service elsewhere.

Schizophrenia Association of Great Britain, Bryn Hyfryd, The Crescent, Bangor, Gwynedd LL57 2AG. Tel. (0248) 354048.

Scottish Association for Mental Health, 40 Shandwick Place, Edinburgh EH2 4RT. Tel. (031) 225 4446.

SML (suppliers of 'artificial daylight' equipment for seasonal affective disorder), Unit 4, Wye Industrial Estate, London Road, High Wycombe, Bucks HP11 1LH. Tel. (0494) 448727.

Women's Equality Group of London Strategic Policy Unit, 20 Vauxhall Bridge Road, London SW1V 2SB. Tel. (01) 633 3643.

SELF-HELP AND MUTUAL HELP ORGANIZATIONS

Accept, 200 Seagrave Road, London SW6 1RQ. Tel. (01) 381 3155. Counselling and psychotherapy for people with dependence problems related to alcohol, illicit drugs and tranquillizers, in eight centres in the London area.

Al-Anon/Alateen, 61 Great Dover Street, London SE1 4YF. Tel. (01) 403 0888. For families of those with drink problems.

Alcohol Concern, 305 Gray's Inn Road, London WC1X 8QF. Tel. (01) 833 3471.

Alcohol Counselling Service, 34 Electric Lane, London SW9 8JT. Tel. (01) 737 3579.

Alcoholics Anonymous, PO Box 514, 11 Redcliffe Gardens, London SW10 9BQ. Tel. (01) 352 9779. See local telephone book for nearest group.

Alzheimer's Disease Society, 3rd Floor, Bank Buildings, Fulham Broadway, London SW6 1EP. Tel. (01) 381 3177.

Anorexia Anonymous, 24 Westmoreland Road, London SW13 9RY. Tel. (01) 748 3994.

Anorexic Aid, 11 Priory Road, High Wycombe, Buckinghamshire. Tel. 0494 21431.

Anorexic Family Aid, Sackville Place, 44 Magdalen Street, Norwich NR3 1JE. Tel. (0603) 621414.

Association for Post-Natal Depression, c/o Queen Charlotte's Hospital, Goldhawk Road, London W6 0XN. Tel. (01) 748 4666.

Breakaway, SCSF Ltd, 57 Garrick Close, London W5 1AT. Tel. (01) 991 2169. Provides wide range of social, cultural and sporting activities for non-cohabiting people aged 23-45 years in Greater London area. Kaleidoscope is a sister organization for older members.

Compassionate Friends, 6 Denmark Street, Bristol BS1 5DQ. Tel. (0272) 292778. Provides counselling and support for bereaved parents.

Crisis Counselling for Alleged Shoplifters, c/o National Consumer Protection Council, London NW4 4NY. Tel. (01) 202 5787 (chairman); (01) 722 3685 (answerphone); (01) 958 8859 (after 7 p.m.).

Cruse (National Organisation for Widows and their Children), 126 Sheen Road, Richmond, Surrey TW9 1UR. Tel. (01) 940 4818/9047.

DAWN (Drugs, Alcohol, Women, Nationally), Omnibus Work Space, 39 North Road, London N7. Tel. (01) 700 4653.

Depressives Anonymous, 36 Chestnut Avenue, Neverley, North Humberside HU17 9QU. Tel. (0482) 860619.

Depressives Associated, PO Box 5, Castletown, Portland, Dorset DT5 1BQ.

Families Anonymous, 88 Caledonian Road, London N1 9DN. Tel. (01) 278 8805. Network of support groups for families of people with drug dependence problems.

Gamblers Anonymous, 17-23 Blantyre Street, Cheyne

Walk, London SW10 0DT. Tel. (01) 352 3060.

GROW – Britain, 2 Tynemouth Street, London SW6 2QT. Tel. (01) 736 0291. Non-denominational 'personal growth' programme based on Twelve Steps of Alcoholics Anonymous.

Manic-Depressive Fellowship, 51 Sheen Road, Richmond, Surrey. Tel. (01) 940 6235.

Meet-a-Mum (MAMA), 3 Woodside Avenue, London SE25 5DW. Tel. (01) 654 3137. Support group to help prevent post-natal depression.

ME (myalgic encephalomyelitis) **Association,** PO Box 8, Stanford-le-Hope, Essex SS17 8EX.

Miscarriage Association, 18 Stoneybrook Close, West Bretton, Wakefield, West Yorkshire WF4 4TP. Tel. (0924) 85515.

Narcotics Anonymous, London SW10. Tel. (01) 351 6794/6066. Telephone for information about local branches for people with drug dependence problems.

National Association for Premenstrual Syndrome, 25 Market Street, Guildford, Surrey GU1 4LB. Tel. (0483) 572806/572715.

National Association for Widows, Stafford & District Voluntary Service, Chell Road, Stafford ST16 2QA. Tel. (0785) 45465.

National Association of Victims Support Schemes, 17a Electric Lane, London SW9 8LA. Tel. (01) 737 2010. Support and advice for victims of crime, with branches throughout country.

National Childbirth Trust, 9 Queensborough Terrace, London W2 3TB. Tel. (01) 221 3833. Network of specialist counsellors who provide help and support for mothers with post-natal and other problems.

National Council for the Divorced and Separated, 13 High Street, Little Shelford, Cambridge CB2 5ES. Tel. (0623) 648297.

National Drinkwatchers Network, 200 Seagrave Road, London SW6 1RQ. Tel. (01) 381 3157. Groups run by Accept for people with mild alcohol problems.

National Federation of Solo Clubs, Room 8, Ruskin Chambers, 119 Corporation Street, Birmingham B4 6RY.

Tel. (021) 236 2879. For unattached people over 25 years of age.

National Stepfamily Association, 162 Tenison Road, Cambridge CB1 2DP. Tel. (0223) 460312 (general inquiries; (0223) 460313 (counselling).

Northern Ireland Agoraphobic Society, 84 University Street, Belfast B17 1HE. Tel. (0232) 228474.

Open Door Association, 447 Pensby Road, Heswall, Merseyside L61 9PQ. Tel. (051) 648 2022. Support and counselling for agoraphobia sufferers.

Outsiders Club, PO Box 4ZB, London W1A 4ZB. Tel. (01) 741 3332/ 958 3681. Offers an opportunity for social life and friendship for people who feel inhibited by emotional problems or physical handicaps.

Parkinson's Disease Society, 36 Portland Place, London W1N 3DG. Tel. (01) 323 1174.

Phobics Society, 4 Cheltenham Road, Chorlton-cum-Hardy, Manchester M21 1QN. Tel. (061) 881 1937.

Portia Trust, 15 Senhouse Street, Maryport, Cumbria CA15 6AB. Tel. (0900) 812 114. Offers counselling by letter or telephone to mentally distressed women accused of crimes such as shoplifting.

Scottish Association of Victims Support Schemes, 7a Royal Terrace, Edinburgh EH7 5AB. Tel. (031) 558 1380.

Stillbirth and Neonatal Death Society, 29-31 Euston Road, London NW1 2SD. Tel. (01) 833 2851.

Tranx, 17 Peel Road, Harrow, Middlesex HA3 7QX. Tel. (01) 427 2065. National advisory and counselling service for people with tranquillizer dependence problems.

Turning Point, 9-12 Long Lane, London EC1A 9HA. Tel. (01) 606 3947. Offers counselling and residential therapy in many areas for people with alcohol and drug abuse problems.

Women's Health Concern, Ground Floor, 17 Earl's Terrace, London W8 6LP. Tel.(01) 602 6669. Advises on problems related to menstruation and the menopause.

Women's Health Information Centre, 52 Featherstone Street, London EC1Y 8RT. Tel. (01) 251 6580. Supplies information on women's self-help and health groups.

Women's Information Referral and Enquiry Service,

PO Box 20, Oxford. Tel. (0865) 240991.

PROFESSIONAL COUNSELLING AND THERAPY
Arbours Association, 41A Weston Park, London N8. Tel. (01) 340 7646. Offers crisis counselling by telephone to callers in distress. Provides analytic and other forms of psychotherapy on a short- or long-term basis; and long- and short-stay residential treatment in therapeutic communities.
Association for Applied Hypnosis, 33-39 Abbey Park Road, Grimsby, South Humberside DN32 0HS. Tel. (0472) 47702. Psychotherapy with hypnosis to relax client or to facilitate positive suggestion techniques.
Association for Family Therapy, 6 Heol Seddon, Danescourt, Llandaff, Cardiff CF5 2QX.
Association for Group and Individual Psychotherapy, 29 St Mark's Crescent, London NW1. Tel. (01) 485 9141. Individual analytically-oriented psychotherapy.
Association for Humanistic Psychology, 62 Southwark Bridge Road, London SE1. Tel. (01) 928 8254. Provides information on sources for Transactional Analysis and a wide range of alternative therapies.
Association of Pastoral Care of the Mentally Ill, 39 St John's Lane, London EC1M 4BJ. Tel. (01) 253 9524.
Association of Sexual and Marital Therapists, PO Box 62, Sheffield S10. Professional association which can advise on the availability of local clinics and therapists.
Behavioural Psychology Services Ltd, 3 Brighton Road, London N2 8JU. Tel. (01) 346 9646. Supplies LifeSkills series of audio cassette tapes and books by behavioural psychologist Dr Robert Sharpe, director of Institute of Behaviour Therapy. Titles include *Assertiveness* (book) and tapes on relaxation, shyness, assertiveness, agoraphobia, etc.
Birmingham Women's Counselling and Therapy Centre, 43 Ladywood Middleway, Birmingham B16 8HA. Tel. (021) 455 8677. Offers free therapy and counselling, using psychoanalytic and humanistic techniques.
Board of Social Responsibility of Church of Scotland, 121 George Street, Edinburgh EH2 4YN. Tel. (031) 225 5722.

Information on pastoral counselling service in Scotland.

British Association for Counselling, 37a Sheep Street, Rugby, Warwickshire CV21 3BX. Tel. (0788) 78328/9. Offers information on services providing professional counselling, and publishes directories listing individual counsellors and counselling agencies.

British Association of Psychotherapists, 121 Hendon Lane, London N3 3PR. Tel. (01) 346 1747. Concerned with training of analytical psychotherapists, and provides an assessment and referral service for clients.

British Homoeopathic Association, 27a Devonshire Street, London W1N 1RJ. Tel. (01) 935 2163. Promotes study of homoeopathy, which involves treating symptoms with minute amounts of substances which in larger amounts could cause similar symptoms. Provides information on practitioners.

British Hypnotherapy Association, 67 Upper Berkeley Square, London W1H 7DH. Tel. (01) 723 4443. Offers analytic psychotherapy using hypnosis to relax client.

British Psychological Society, 48 Princess Road East, Leicester LE1 7DR. Tel. (0533) 549568. A learned society of psychologists. Cannot provide names of individual members. Directs inquirers to chairman of their regional health authority.

British Society of Medical and Dental Hypnosis, PO Box 6, 42 Links Road, Ashtead, Surrey KT21 2HT. Tel. (03722) 73522.

Camden Psychotherapy Unit, 25-31 Tavistock Place, London WC1H 9SE. Tel. (01) 388 2071 ext 48. Offers analytic psychotherapy. Free to Camden residents.

Catholic Marriage Advisory Council, 15 Lansdowne Road, London W11 3AJ. Tel. (01) 727 0141.

Centre for Advancement of Counselling, 56C Hale Lane, London NW7 3PR. Tel. (01) 959 8084, 24-hour service. Specializes in counselling training for staff working with cancer and AIDS patients.

Churches' Council for Health and Healing, St Marylebone Parish Church, Marylebone Road, London NW1 5LT. Tel. (01) 486 9644. Information available on services.

Church of England Board for Social Responsibility,

Church House, Great Smith Street, London SW1. Tel.
(01) 222 9011. Can provide information on C of E
counselling services throughout the country.

Clinic of Psychotherapy, Garden Flat, 26 Belsize Square,
London NW3. Tel. (01) 903 6455. Offers analytic
psychotherapy. Initial assessments by medical staff.

Contact, 2a Ribble Street, Newtownards Road, Belfast. Tel.
(0232) 57848. Offers counselling to adolescents and
young adults on a walk-in basis or by telephone.

Family Welfare Association, 501 Kingsland Road, London
E8 4AU. Tel. (01) 254 6251. Counselling provided by
social workers for individuals, couples and families, in 12
centres based in London, Milton Keynes and North-
ampton.

Group Analytic Practice, 88 Montagu Mansions, London
W1H 1LF. Tel. (01) 935 3103/3085. Offers analytic
psychotherapy to groups.

Institute for Complementary Medicine, 2 Portland Place,
London W1N 2AF. Tel. (01) 636 9543. Information on
alternative treatments such as acupuncture.

Institute of Behaviour Therapy, 38 Queen Anne Street,
London W1M 9LB. Tel. (01) 580 4972. Private treatment
provided by three consultants who specialize in
behaviour and cognitive therapy for clients with
problems such as phobias, compulsions and relationship
difficulties. See also Behavioural Psychology Services
Ltd.

Institute of Group Analysis, 1 Daleham Gardens, London
NW3 5BY. Tel. (01) 431 2693. Offers psychoanalytically-
based group therapy.

Institute of Psychoanalysis, 63 New Cavendish Street, W1.
Tel. (01) 580 4952.

Institute of Psychotherapy and Social Studies, 5 Lake
House, London NW3 2SH. Tel. (01) 794 4147. Training
and treatment centre with integrated analytic and
humanistic approach.

Isis Centre, 43 Little Clarendon Street, Oxford OX1 2HU.
Tel. (0865) 56648. Offers professional counselling on an
individual and family basis under NHS for Oxfordshire
residents.

Jewish Marriage Council, 23 Ravenshurst Avenue, London NW4. Tel. (01) 203 6311.

Leeds Women's Counselling and Therapy Service, Top Floor, Oxford Chambers, Oxford Place, Leeds LS1 3AX. Tel. (0532) 455725. Offers psychoanalytic, humanistic and cognitive therapies where appropriate to client's needs.

Lincoln Clinic and Institute for Psychotherapy, 77 Westminster Bridge Road, London SE1 7HS. Tel. (01) 928 7211/261 9236. Training and treatment centre offering analytic therapy and shorter-term 'focal psychotherapy' which focuses on specific problems.

London Centre for Psychotherapy, 19 Fitzjohn's Avenue, London NW3 5JY. Tel. (01) 435 0873. Training and treatment centre with analytical orientation. Clients assessed by medically qualified therapist before treatment.

London Youth Advisory Centre, 26 Prince of Wales Road, London NW5 3LG. Tel. (01) 467 4792. Offers counselling and psychotherapy to people aged from 13 to 25 years of age.

Maisner Centre, 57a Church Road, Hove, East Sussex BN3 2BD. Tel. (0273) 729818/29334. Private clinic specializing in treatment of bulimia and compulsive eating.

Maudsley Hospital, Denmark Hill, London SE5 8AZ. Tel. (01) 703 6333. Leading NHS psychiatric hospital. Patients seen on GP referral. Also 24-hour, seven days a week, emergency clinic, where patients in urgent need of help are seen without appointment and without medical referral.

Nafsiyat, The Inter-Cultural Therapy Centre, 278 Seven Sisters Road, London N4 2HY. Tel. (01) 263 4130. Short- and long-term treatment using analytic approach and with special consideration of cultural factors. Free to Islington residents, fee charged to clients from other areas.

National Association of Young People's Counselling and Advisory Services, 17-23 Albion Street, Leicester LE1 6GD. Tel. (0533) 554775 (ext. 22 & 36).

National Marriage Guidance Council, Herbert Gray

College, Little Church Street, Rugby, Warwickshire. Tel.
(0788) 73241.

North London Centre for Group Therapy, 6b Priory Close,
London N14 4AW. Tel. (01) 440 1451. Offers psychoanalytically-based group therapy.

Relaxation for Living, 29 Burwood Park Road, Walton-on-
Thames, Surrey KT12 5LH. Registered charity with
classes in many areas. Supplies leaflets and cassette
tapes, including Dr Claire Weekes' relaxation programmes. Large s.a.e. for details.

School of Hypnosis and Advanced Psychotherapy, 28
Finsbury Park Road, London N4 2JX. Tel. (01) 359 6991,
24-hour answering service. Professional training
courses.

Scottish Institute of Human Relations, 56 Albany Street,
Edinburgh. Tel. (031) 556 6454. Members – some
working in Glasgow – offer psychoanalytically-based
therapy.

Scottish Marriage Guidance Council, 26 Frederick Street,
Edinburgh EH2 2JR. Tel. (031) 225 5006.

South London Psychotherapy Group, 19 Broom Water,
Teddington, Middlesex TW11 9QT. Tel. (01) 977 6303.
Offers analytic psychotherapy.

Tavistock Clinic, 120 Belsize Lane, London NW3 5BA. Tel.
(01) 435 7111. Leading training centre for psychoanalytic
psychotherapists. Offers therapy under the National
Health Service. Its Young People's Counselling Service
offers help on a self-referral basis to people aged from 16
to 30 years.

UK Training College of Hypnotherapy and Counselling,
10 Alexander Street, London W2 5NT. Tel. (01) 221 1796
& 727 2006. Professional training courses held in
London, Bristol, Ireland and Scotland. Emphasis on use
of self-hypnosis for personal growth and assertiveness
training.

Westminster Pastoral Foundation, 23 Kensington Square,
London W8 5HN. Tel. (01) 937 6956. Offers individual,
family and marital counselling on a non-denominational
basis. Information provided on affiliated centres
throughout the country.

Women's Therapy Centre, 6 Manor Gardens, London N7 6LA. Tel. (01) 263 6200. Offers analytically-oriented individual and group therapy, and a range of other techniques as appropriate for different clients. The centre also specializes in treating clients with eating problems.

Young People's Counselling Service (see Tavistock Clinic).

Select bibliography

Asso, Doreen. *The Real Menstrual Cycle* (John Wiley 1983)

Berne, Eric. *Games People Play* (Transactional Analysis) (Penguin 1970)

Blair, Pat. *Know Your Medicines* (Age Concern 1986)

Brandon, Althea & David. *Consumers as Colleagues* (MIND pamphlet 1987)

Brown, Dennis & Jonathan Pedder. *Introduction to Psychotherapy* (Tavistock Publications 1979)

Brown, George & Tirril Harris. *Social Origins of Depression* (Tavistock Publications 1978)

Brown, Paul & Carolyn Faulder. *Treat Yourself to Sex* (Penguin 1979)

Byrne, Pat & Barrie Long. *Doctors Talking to Patients* (Royal College of General Practitioners 1984)

Chernin, Kim. *Womansize: the tyranny of slenderness* (Women's Press 1983)

Clare, Anthony. *Psychiatry in Dissent* (Tavistock Publications 1976)

Cochrane, Raymond. *The Social Creation of Mental Illness* (Longman 1983)

Comport, Maggie. *Towards Happy Motherhood: Understanding Post-natal Depression* (Corgi 1987)

Dally, Peter & Joan Gomez. *Anorexia Nervosa* (William Heinemann 1979)

Dickson, Anne. *A Woman in Your Own Right: Assertiveness and You* (Quartet 1982)

Duckworth, Tessa & David Miller. *Flying Without Fear* (Sheldon Press 1983)

Emerson, Joyce & Clare Marc Wallace. *Schizophrenia* (British Medical Association 1969)

Fraser, Antonia. *The Weaker Vessel* (Methuen 1984)

Fry, Anthony. *Safe Space* (J M Dent 1987)

Gavron, Hannah. *The Captive Wife* (Routledge & Kegan Paul 1966)

Gibbs, Angelina. *Understanding Mental Health* (Consumers' Association/Hodder & Stoughton 1986)

Haddon, Celia. *Women and Tranquillisers* (Sheldon Press 1984)

Jennings, Sue (ed). *Creative Therapy* (Pitman 1975)

Jones, Kathleen. *History of the Mental Health Services* (Routledge & Kegan Paul 1976)

Kelly, Desmond. *A Practical Handbook for the Treatment of Depression* (Parthenon 1987)

———— (ed.), with Richard France and David Burns. *Feeling Good* (Signet 1980)

Knight, Lindsay. *Talking to a Stranger* (Fontana 1986)

Kovel, Joel. *A Complete Guide to Therapy* (Penguin 1978)

Lacey, R. & S. Woodward. *That's Life survey on tranquillisers* (BBC Publications 1985)

Lake, Tony. *Living With Grief* (Sheldon Press 1984)

Lawrence, Marilyn. *The Anorexic Experience* (Women's Press 1984)

Levete, Gina. *The Creative Tree* (Michael Russell Publishing, Salisbury, Wilts. 1987)

Lewis, David. *Fight Your Phobia – and Win* (Sheldon Press 1984)

Lum, Claude. *Modern Trends in Psychosomatic Medicine Vol. 3* (Butterworth 1976)

MacLeod, Sheila. *The Art of Starvation: anorexia observed* (Virago Press 1981)

Mackarness, Richard. *Not All in the Mind* (Pan 1976)

Mama, Amina, Maria Mars, Prue Stevenson. *Breaking the Silence: Women's Imprisonment* (Women's Equality Group/ London Strategic Policy Unit 1987)

Marks, Isaac. *Living with Fear* (McGraw-Hill 1979)

McConville, Brigid. *Women Under the Influence* (Virago Press 1983)

McKeon, Patrick. *Coping with Depression and Elation* (Sheldon Press 1986)

Melville, Joy. *Phobias and Obsessions* (George Allen & Unwin 1977)

———— *The Tranquilliser Trap* (Fontana 1984)

Moss, Linda. *Art for Health's Sake* (1987). Available from Department of Architecture, Manchester Polytechnic, Loxford Tower, Lower Chatham Street, Manchester M15 6HA

Murgatroyd, Stephen. *Counselling and Helping* (Methuen 1986)

Neuman, Fredric. *Fighting Fear* (David & Charles 1986)

Nairne, Kathy & Gerrilyn Smith. *Dealing with Depression* (Women's Press 1984)

Nicholson, John. *Men and Women: how different are they?* (Oxford University Press 1984)

Oakley, Ann. *The Sociology of Housework* (Martin Robertson 1974)

O'Faolain, Julia and Lauro Martines (eds). *Not in God's Image* (Fontana 1974)

Orbach, Susie. *Fat is a Feminist Issue* (Hamlyn 1978)
————— *Understanding Women* (Penguin 1982)
————— *Hunger Strike* (Faber and Faber 1986)

Peckham, Audrey. *A Woman in Custody* (Fontana 1985)

Parkes, Colin Murray. *Bereavement* (Penguin 1975)

Pietroni, Patrick. *Holistic Living* (J M Dent 1986)

Priest, Robert. *Anxiety and Depression* (Martin Dunitz 1983)

Rodway, Avril. *Taking over: how to cope with your elderly parents* (Columbus Books 1987)

Rowe, Dorothy. *The Experience of Depression* (John Wiley 1978)

Royal College of Physicians. *A Great and Growing Evil* (Tavistock Publications 1987)

Royal College of Psychiatrists. *Alcohol and Alcoholism* (Tavistock Publications 1979)

Sanders, Deidre. *Women and Depression* (Sheldon Press 1984)

Saunders, Cicely & Thomas D. Walsh, in *Geigy Pharmaceuticals Bulletin No. 12* (1984)

Sharpe, Robert. *LifeSkills 1: Assertiveness* (Behavioural Psychology Services Ltd)

Showalter, Elaine. *The Female Malady: women, madness and English Culture 1830–1980* (Virago Press 1987)

Shreeve, Caroline. *Depression* (Turnstone 1984)

Stanway, Andrew. *Overcoming Depression* (Hamlyn 1983)

Stern, Richard. *Behavioural Techniques* (Academic Press 1978)

Stern, Vivien. *Bricks of Shame: Britain's Prisons* (Penguin 1987)

Sutherland, Stuart. *Breakdown* (Granada 1977)

Taylor, F. Kraupl. *Psychopathology: its causes and symptoms* (Butterworth 1966)

Thompson, Keith. *Caring for an Elderly Relative: a guide to home care* (Martin Dunitz 1986)

Trauer, Tom. *Coping with Stress* (Salamander Books 1986)

Tyrer, P. *How to stop taking tranquillisers* (Sheldon Press 1986)

Watts, A. G. (ed). *Counselling at Work* (Bedford Square Press 1977)

Weekes, Claire. *Self-Help for your Nerves* (Angus & Robertson 1985)

———— *Relaxation for Living* (Angus & Robertston 1985)

Westland, Pamela. *All in a Good Cause* (Columbus Books 1986)

Wilson, Judy. *Self-Help Groups* (Longman 1987)

Women in MIND group. *Finding Our Own Solutions* (MIND 1986)

Yaffé, Maurice. *Taking the Fear out of Flying* (David & Charles 1987)

Zimbardo, Philip G. *Shyness* (Addison-Wesley 1977)

Index